In Praise of *End Dieting Hell*

"Michelle is passionate and wise surrounding this topic. I highly recommend this book that will change your perspective, life and waist line. Working with her has always been high quality and now she has put this into a book."

—**Dr. D. Lindsey Berkson**, Best-selling Author of *Safe Hormones, Smart Women; Sexy Brain, Dr. Berkson's Best Health Radio and Membership with Hangouts and Q&A,* drlindseyberkson.com

"This book is a breath of fresh air for those who struggle with their weight. Readers will discover new science-based insights to help them shift from frustration, shame, guilt and hopelessness to relief, understanding, and peace with their weight and body image."

—**Dr. Ritamarie Loscalzo**, MS, DC, CCN, DACBN, Founder of the Institute of Nutritional Endocrinology, https://drritamarie.com

"Michelle brings a whole new approach to an old problem that plagues most of the population. This is a must read if you're ready to end dieting hell!"

—*Jill Lublin*, *International Speaker and 4x Best-selling Author,* JillLublin.com

"Michelle Melendez provides valuable insights about the emotional roots behind weight loss. When you get to the emotional core behind your struggle, you are finally free to live the life you've always wanted. Michelle shows you what you most need to know — how to move through the emotional trap and into a body you love."

—**Misa Hopkins**, Best-selling Author of *The Root of All Healing*

"Michelle beautifully explains how your body is emotionally addicted to struggling with your weight. It really is revolutionary information! This book is an inspiration and insightful new approach to a painful topic and chronic problem."

—**Dr. Julie Wilkening**, DC, CSCS,
Functional Medicine & Habit Change
Practitioner, www.DrJulieWilkening.com

"The most important journey we can take is that of self-love, and learning to love our bodies is a significant part of that. With vulnerability and wisdom, Michelle illuminates this path and helps us come to a deeper understanding of our own emotional addictions and how to free ourselves from them."

—**Tricia Nelson**, Best-selling Author of *Heal Your Hunger: 7 Simple Steps to End Emotional Eating Now*

"End Dieting Hell is a Must Read... the perfect guidebook for anyone struggling with excess weight and a negative body image. Filled with wisdom, Michelle Melendez leaves the reader with much-needed hope and a roadmap for discovering a body they can love."

—**Debora Wayne**, The Pain Free Living Program®

"This book will give you new understandings of why you've struggled with weight for so long. Michelle serves up golden nuggets of science-based wisdom that is rarely, if ever, explained. It's a perfect book for anyone who is ready to live in a body they love."

—**Louise Jeffrey**, Nutritional Therapist
Trained in Traditional Chinese Medicine,
Strategic Psychotherapy, Clinical Hypnotherapy,
and Dynamic Eating Psychology

End Dieting Hell

*How to find peace with your
body and release the weight*

MICHELLE MELENDEZ

Creator of the *Live in a Body You Love*[TM] *program*
and Founder of *Women Being Fit*

End Dieting Hell
Published by Michelle Melendez
Kealakekua, Hawaii 96750

Library of Congress Control Number: 2019907493
ISBN: 978-0-578-52698-0

Cover Design by Manuel Amaro
Cover Photos by Ralph Gibbs
Illustrations by Usman Rafique
Interior Design by Miguel Kilantang
Editing by Jennifer Jas & Lori Spaeth

FIRST EDITION

www.michellemelendezauthor.com

Printed in the United States of America.

DEDICATION

This book is dedicated to any person who has ever felt hopeless, ashamed, embarrassed or frustrated with their weight. It's time for peace. You deserve that!

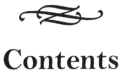

Contents

Acknowledgments

I want to acknowledge my sister, Rebecca Melendez, and dear friend, Benji Quigley, for putting up with my long hours at the computer to complete this book.

Thank you to all my new and old friends for being patient every time we had plans and I needed to cancel to finish this book.

Thank you, Denise Lindsey, for always being so inspiring every time I said, "The book is done!" Ha! Guess what? It's finally done!

Thank you, Mom, for listening to all my health advice even when you didn't want to. I appreciate how you always accept me the way I am. I love you.

Thank you, Steve Diggs, founder of NYSA Therapy, for all your advice on human behavior and how to create lasting change. You are making a huge difference in the world.

Thank you to all my clients for sharing their lives and letting me explore with them their painful journeys struggling with weight. Also, for giving me permission to share some of your stories in this book. I am so inspired by you. Thank you for not giving up and for taking my guidance to heart to create a new life in a body you love. It has meant a lot to me to be there with you.

Thank you, Lori Spaeth, Sara Rogers, Carol Matson, Ellen Petrill, Tess Byler, Elena Shea, Teena James and all of the Pilates Full Body members. Without your participation in my program I wouldn't have had the time to write this book.

Thank you, Jill Lublin, for teaching me so much about the publishing world. I couldn't have done this without you.

Thank you, Jon Lovgren, author of *"The Magic Words,"* for all your advice and video help. You inspired me to complete this book when it was sitting on the shelf!

Thank you, Jennifer Jas, editor and founder of *Words With Jas LLC*. I appreciate your patience and your guidance to make this book what it is today!

Thank you, Lori Spaeth for saying, "Yes" to editing this book at the last minute. Words can't express how much I appreciate you.

Thank you to all my colleagues who wrote a testimonial for this book and for helping me spread the word!

Thank you, Manuel Amaro, Usman Rafique and Miguel Kilantang for the many edits you did that went beyond our final drafts. I so appreciate you.

Thank you, Ralph Gibbs for taking my headshots and turning the experience into a fun photoshoot. I had no idea the spontaneous picture of me with my arms out would be the cover of my first published book.

Thank you, reader, for choosing this book and taking your next step to find peace with your body and to release the weight. By doing so, you will help make the world a better place, and we are all ready for that.

Introduction

Why should you listen to me?

If you're reading this, you've probably been struggling with your weight for years or even most of your life. You've been on tons of diets and probably, at least once, hired a fitness trainer, dietitian or both.

You're frustrated and tired of trying to lose weight… AGAIN!

Guess what? I have never struggled with my weight.

If that turns you off, I understand. Here is something that may turn you back on again and make you want to take a seat and immediately start reading Chapter One.

I have been a fitness trainer since 1996. I discovered something that I never learned in the fitness industry or after becoming a weight-loss specialist. It's the key to why you struggle with your weight and it is the reason why most people will go their entire lives NEVER living in a body they love.

Are you ready for this?

You are cellularly and emotionally addicted to the feeling of struggling with your weight, and that addiction sabotages your weight-loss efforts.

Yes, I said, "ADDICTED." Does that sound crazy?

I was floored when I learned this, because I had been trying to find the answer as to why many of my clients yo-yoed with their weight even after I coached them and they successfully lost weight. If that describes you, there's a reason you found this book.

Are you a professional dieter? Then you know dieting can be HELL!

It is super painful to be successful for a short time on a diet and then go back to where you started, or worse… you gain even MORE weight! That rollercoaster ride damages your self-confidence, self-love and outlook on life. You resent other people who have maintained their weight loss and women who have never had to deal with it in the first place.

You feel angry, frustrated, embarrassed and ashamed, and ask questions like, *"Why is this so hard?!"* It might even feel like maybe you're supposed to be fat.

I'm here to tell you that is NOT your fate!

There is a reason your journey has been so hard and you will never find the answer in a diet or exercise program, because it simply hasn't yet been taught in that way. The industry doesn't know about this.

I learned this material outside the fitness industry when I started studying quantum physics and cellular communication. That's when I knew I had hit gold and could finally help my clients the way I wanted to.

From what I learned, I created the *Live in a Body You Love*™ three-month program. This book is based on those teachings. During that program, my clients join me on the Big Island of Hawaii for a seven-day retreat where they swim with dolphins, snorkel with manta rays, hike the volcano and let the healing energy of the island bring them peace. It's a life-changing experience that I hope you will join me on someday.

For now, let this book be the catalyst that ends dieting hell and starts you on an emotional expansion toward love and forgiveness of yourself and others. I know you can do this!

Get ready to understand the science behind how *emotional expansion* works to create change and move you toward a body you love. I'm so excited to share this with you. I have included practices that will support you to release your emotional addictions. I recommend that you read through the entire book once before trying a practice. Let this new info sink in. Then, read it again and try each practice as soon as you read it. When you find one that tugs your heartstrings, BINGO! Add it to your daily routine and use it! Your heart will tell you which ones are right for you. Trust it! Even add an alarm to your cell phone to remind you to do the practice daily.

I'm thrilled you have chosen my book to help you. You deserve to have peace in your body! It's time!

Mahalo.

My Story

I want to share my story so you understand why I'm so passionate about this work even though I have never struggled with my weight. When I was thirteen years old, I found out I had a slight case of scoliosis. Scoliosis is where part of your back is curved, and in my case, the right side of my back sits slightly behind the left. It wasn't bad enough that I had to wear a back brace, and I was grateful for that.

However, one of my breasts was larger than the other, and being a thirteen-year-old… I was horrified.

I Hated My Body!

I felt embarrassed, ashamed, humiliated and completely insecure. This was especially the case if cute guys were checking me out. I was sure they could tell my boobs were uneven and I was afraid they would laugh at me.

One night, my nightmare came true! I was making out with a guy, and he started touching my breasts. Then he started laughing. I was mortified! I didn't know what to do so I acted like nothing happened and kept kissing him. Luckily, my sister showed up and we promptly left.

I remember my thoughts as I looked in the mirror: "Why me? Why did this happen to me?"

Buying new clothes was emotionally painful. Every time I was in the fitting room of a department store trying on new clothes, I would slowly open the door to look out and make sure the fitting room attendant wasn't around. I didn't want anyone to see what I looked like before I had the chance to make sure that my uneven breasts were not noticeable.

Before my sister and I went out, I would ask her the same question every time, *"Can you tell?"* She knew what that meant: *Can you tell that one boob is larger than the other?* She always had the same answer: *"No, Michelle. You can't tell and no one is going to care anyway!"*

Well, I could tell, so I normally still felt ashamed and went back to my room to change clothes or get a sweater to cover my body.

I remember being at school one day and seeing a friend who was toned and looked amazing! Her name was Angela and she told me she worked out three times a week. I thought, *I'm going to start working out! I bet that would fix things.* My goal was to only workout the larger side of my chest, so it would tone up and hopefully shrink down, and then my boobs would look even. Sounds silly now, but back then it made total sense!

Something happened when I started working out that I wasn't expecting… I started to have more energy, sleep better and feel somewhat better about myself regardless of my uneven boobs. I was hooked!

I finished high school and decided not to go to college right away. I wanted to "find myself." After an adventure in L.A. and back home again within six months, I ended up in San Luis Obispo, California, needing a job. As luck would have it, a gym was hiring. The owner needed instructors and would pay for anyone interested in getting certified to teach various exercise modalities. I was in! I learned to teach Body Pump (a toning class), Martial Fitness Kickboxing, Reebok Spin, Pilates and many others. I also got my personal training certification.

Once I hit my thirties, I had been a fitness trainer for ten years with almost twelve fitness certifications under my belt. Surprisingly, I still struggled with my body image. What I didn't understand was that the actions I was taking to get fit and to be a trainer weren't reconditioning the emotional vibrational energy that my body was addicted to. Oh, it helped. I felt strong and at times, very confident — especially when I was teaching group exercise classes, which I still love doing. However, going out was the same story. I'd wear shirts and dresses that didn't show the unevenness of my breasts, or I'd pad the right side of my bra to make them look even.

I was sick of feeling ashamed, frustrated and humiliated by my body, even though it was fit and toned. I finally decided to do something radically different. I signed up for a *Creating a Better Body Image* program.

I remember a particular practice I had to do that was *VERY* uncomfortable. The practice involved doing a striptease for myself in the mirror. I was so uncomfortable doing this, even though I was at home by myself. I didn't want to look at my body in the mirror because I knew I wouldn't like what I saw. Then I decided if I was going to do this, I had to make it fun. So I lit candles and turned on fun music, and slowly took off my clothes and stared at myself. I saw the cellulite on my legs, the unevenness of my boobs and even a bit of a poochy belly.

Part of the practice was to consciously feel something different, so I started to think about what could be different.

Then, something came over me…

I thought about the many miles my legs had walked, and all the people my arms had hugged, and the strangers' hands my hands had shaken who often became close friends — and relief came over me. The feeling of relief and appreciation consumed me. What I didn't know at the time was that I was shifting the emotional vibrational energy that had been held in every cell of my body most of my life.

I decided to practice this new feeling every day in the mirror for two to five minutes, and that's when change truly began to happen.

Had you told me in my thirties that I would be writing a book in my forties and disclosing the unevenness of my breasts, I would have told you… *YOU'RE CRAZY!* I was so ashamed of my body. I didn't want ANYONE to know about it, EVER!

Today, I literally feel so differently about my body that I don't mind sharing the truth of how I felt. I even did a live spoken-word performance and revealed my ENTIRE self-loathing story onstage to about sixty-plus friends and strangers. You can watch it by going to: http://womenbeingfit.com/michelles-story/

If you have been struggling with your weight most of your life, your ego wants you to be fat. It has tricked you into thinking you are someone who struggles with your weight and it wants you to stay that way. I'm here to tell you that is NOT who you are. That is only a **memorized addictive pattern** in the over fifty to seventy-trillion cells of your body, and you can release it!

Let me explain…

CHAPTER ONE

Your Ego Wants You to Be Fat

If you have struggled with your weight for years, your brain and body have **memorized how to live in a body you don't love,** and you repeat those thoughts, actions and emotions daily.

Your ego has tricked you into believing your thoughts and actions are who you are. They ARE NOT who you are! They are only memorized ways of being that you are emotionally addicted too. It feels normal and familiar in your body to struggle with your weight.

The key phrase is: "It feels NORMAL!"

Let me give you an example.

Conference Story

I once had a booth at a women's conference, and I remember a lady walking down the aisle toward me. As soon as she saw me, she said, "No, no I don't want to talk about exercise!" I looked at her, smiled, and said, "That's great! Do you know you're emotionally addicted to ignoring exercise?" She paused, stared at me for a moment and asked what I meant. I asked her to tell me why she didn't want to talk about exercise.

She said she had an exercise room in her home that she walked by every day, even though she knew she should go in and exercise.

I asked her how many times she had told someone that story of her exercise room that she never used. She said that she tells that story all the time. I then asked her how she feels when she walks past the room, knowing she should go in and exercise. She told me that she feels frustrated and guilty.

I revealed to her that those feelings were emotional addictions in her body and that she felt normal walking past her exercise room feeling that way and not going in to workout. If she went in to exercise, it would actually feel weird and probably even wrong. She looked at me and paused again, then said, *"Yeah. You're right."*

If you can relate to that story, then you have emotional addictions that keep you struggling with your weight year after year. The feeling of struggling with your weight is a conditioned addiction in every cell of your body and feels normal even though you don't like it.

This emotional addiction will sabotage every diet or exercise program you go on. In fact, if you lose weight, immediately you feel afraid that you'll gain it back again. One reason for this is you don't know who you would be if you didn't struggle with your weight. Sound familiar?

Not struggling with your weight is foreign to you. You probably can't even picture it and that alone will keep you struggling year after year.

Your emotional addiction too struggling with your weight was created a long time ago. Your brain created it as a memorized pattern to help you cope with an intense experience in your past. If you've struggled with your weight most of your life, then the emotional addiction was created when you were a child. If you started struggling later in life, it was created when you were a teenager or maybe young adult.

Here's a shocker… if you've struggled with your weight your entire life AND your mother and/or father struggled with their weight, the emotional addiction may be ancestral, which means the emotional energy was transferred to you and wasn't created by you. Think of it like a mother who is addicted to heroin. She has a baby addicted to heroin because the chemicals of heroin are passing through her blood and into the fetus. Emotions are chemicals and also transferred to the baby through blood, as well as through energy. For instance, if the emotional addiction started with your father then it was passed to you energetically and not through your blood. This is how you become your parents.

Crazy! I thought it was.

Emotional addictions can be even further back, coming from a grandparent, great-grandparent or even earlier. Emotional energy can be ancestral because energy has no boundaries. It never dies. If an emotional addiction is strong like fear or anger, that energy can move into the next generation.

I believe one of the most amazing things about this work is that when you heal yourself of your emotional conditioning, it can heal your ancestors. It doesn't matter if they are alive or have passed on. You are the evolution of your family, and when you emotionally heal, it goes through your ancestral line. That is one reason why your soul wanted to be a part of your family unit. It's no accident you were born into the family you were born into. I'll explain more about these ideas later.

Let's go back to understanding your emotional addiction, because it is crucial to your success of living in a body you love!

No matter where the emotional addiction came from, if you are addicted to the feeling of struggling with your weight, it is in every cell of your body, and going on a diet or exercise program is not your answer.

Here is how emotional addiction works: As soon as you get up in the morning, **your body sends a signal** to your brain to think thoughts that create the familiar emotional vibration you feel every day.

Do you get on the scale first thing in the morning feeling worried about what it will say?

Do you have a negative thought when you first look in the mirror?

Do you feel embarrassed, ashamed or frustrated with how you look before you leave the house?

That all creates the same emotions that you feel day in and day out, which create the same behaviors and will forever keep you trying to lose weight, and failing!

Here are **clues** to know if you are emotionally addicted to the feeling of struggling with your weight:

- You think about your weight every day.
- You sabotage yourself when you start to lose weight.
- It feels familiar to dislike your body and struggle with your weight.
- You feel like a failure with your weight.
- If you don't get on the scale in the morning, you feel anxious and fearful you've gained weight.

- When you lose weight, you are immediately afraid you'll gain it back.
- You feel ashamed, embarrassed, guilty, frustrated and hopeless when it comes to your weight.
- You don't like having your picture taken, looking in the mirror or being fully seen.

If these sound familiar, your body is emotionally addicted to keeping you struggling with your weight for the *rest of your life!* In fact, your ego will fight to keep this identity alive.

Participant Story

At one of my "Live In A Body You Love" retreats I told a participant that she was not someone who struggled with her weight but someone who was addicted to the feelings and behaviors of struggling with her weight. She actually got angry and told me that she had struggled with her weight most of her life and that is who she was. Her ego was so attached to that identity that she didn't want to believe that wasn't her.

The concept that she wasn't someone who struggled with her weight was foreign to her. When she finally understood that it was only memorized emotional addictive feelings and behaviors that kept her overweight, relief and hope came over her. That started her journey toward new, memorized emotions and ways of being that led to freedom and peace with her body.

Your ego has a stake in you struggling with your weight and it will not want to change. That is how it knows how to behave in your everyday life. Your actions, words and thoughts are of someone who struggles with their weight. If you didn't, you wouldn't know how to behave. There is no behavioral memory patterns of you not struggling with your weight. Your entire identity is based on your struggle! It is who you know yourself to be and it is who other people know you to be, which keeps you believing that is who you are.

Your Ego Does Not Like The Unknown

Your ego doesn't know the everyday thoughts, behaviors and actions it would create if you weren't struggling with your weight. *This is a HUGE reason you self-sabotage.*

It's crucial for you to start exploring who you would be if you were living in a body you love — otherwise, you will never get there. If you don't know what you will be doing, eating, behaving and feeling when you're living in a body you love, how can it happen?

It's like thinking of moving to an amazing, new place. You think it will be great and you dream about it, but instead of exploring what you'll do for money, where you'll live, what establishments you'll enjoy, and planning the date you'll move it stays a dream and nothing changes.

Try this practice and explore who you would be if you didn't struggle with your weight. See how it makes you feel. This may be challenging because it's a new way of thinking about yourself, and that is the whole point! Are you brave enough to give it a try?

Practice: Who Would You Be?

Get a journal and for five to ten minutes, free write anything that comes up after this statement: "If I lived in a body I loved, I would…"

What will your morning routine look like?

How will you feel about yourself?

What will you be saying to yourself?

What will others be saying to you?

What activities will you be doing?

What will your evening routine look like? How will you feel about yourself at the end of the day?

When you get triggered by past traumas, what will you do to be kind and support yourself?

Do this practice for thirty nights before you go to bed, and see what happens.

WARNING: Do not write, *"I would not do..."* That is your body trying to go back to what it knows. Do this practice ONLY stating the positive of what you would be doing. This is challenging and will feel different. That tells you you're on the right track! Oh yeah!

Notice how you feel after this free-writing practice. That feeling can turn into your new normal and it can change everything for you. It's important to do this practice consistently for at least *thirty days,* and I invite you to do it for the rest of your life as a daily practice to create what you want.

Without knowing it, every day you've practiced being someone who's struggled with weight. It's time to practice learning who you would be if you lived in a body you love. You deserve that.

The truth is that you're comfortable in your body and the emotions of struggling with your weight. You may not like it, but it's familiar. It's what you know and how you see yourself. Your ego feels safe with you being right where you are. If you don't rock the boat with ideas of becoming someone else, then all is emotionally well, even though you're not happy. You are safe and your ego gets to be content with the familiarity of what it knows, but you are still not living in a body you love.

I know you want to become someone else or you wouldn't be reading this. I was the same way.

DMV Story

In my teens, my ego told me I was an angry person. I was annoyed with everything all the time and I was miserable. One day, I was coming out of the DMV completely irritated with everyone who worked there and with the whole system.

I looked up at a guy walking toward me with a snarl on my face and he laughed at me. I was totally taken aback. It actually made me stop and notice the present moment.

I looked around and saw that no one else was angry or looked annoyed. I even started to feel a bit ridiculous. Then, for the briefest moment, I recognized that the world didn't revolve around me, which, for being a teenager, was quite an outstanding recognition. I understood that my anger was coming from my need to be right and didn't have anything to do with anyone else.

I then wondered if I really needed to be right and if I could feel something besides anger. I didn't know it at the time, but that moment of being laughed at was what's called a state-change and created a shift in my emotions. It also planted the seed of change in who I thought I was.

Do you need to be right about your struggle with weight? Is it important that you prove to yourself, over and over, how diet and exercise programs don't work for you? What if you could feel something different — what would it be?

As you can see this is not a diet and exercise book. I'm going to take you on a journey that will end dieting hell if that is what you desire. However, this journey is not for everyone. Most people will not want to change their memorized feelings, thoughts and behaviors because they are so addicted to them. Becoming free and learning to live in a body they love is more uncomfortable than holding on to the familiar. Their identities are wrapped up in those feelings. They can't believe they could be someone else, but they can.

Your first step is to see where you are going and what you will be doing when you get there. Then, have compassion for yourself and everything you've been through. There will be tears, anger, sorrow and more joy and relief than you've experienced so far in your life.

Are you willing to take the journey? Let's do it together.

CHAPTER TWO

Why New Year's Resolutions NEVER Work

This chapter will help you understand the science behind how your brain and body work together to keep you overweight, even though that is not what you want.

When you have a feeling, the chemicals and frequency of that feeling leave your brain and enter the cells of your body through a bridge called a receptor site. Each receptor site is created specifically for a different feeling. The more you feel a feeling, the more you create receptor sites that allow that feeling to enter the cells. The more receptor sites you have for a certain feeling, the stronger it is in your body.

Think about the last time you were really angry at someone. That feeling wasn't only in your head; you felt it throughout your entire body. Your body was vibrating at the frequency of anger and it had chemicals that matched it. The same is true for every emotion you've ever felt. Take love for instance. When you're in love, it feels like you're floating on air. Your entire body vibrates at that higher frequency and you feel GREAT!

Emotions can be measured as energetic frequencies. Love and peace are the highest emotional frequencies that exist. That is why you have so much energy. The feeling of love is the vibrational frequency of creation, so when you are feeling love, you are aligned with where your soul came from. That is the reason it feels so good.

Depression is the lowest emotional frequency that exists. You want to sleep when you feel depressed; you have no energy. It is also the furthest emotion from where your soul came from and that is why it feels so bad. All of the other emotions you feel are vibrationally in-between love and depression.

Every two months, your cells divide and the newly created cells duplicate the number of receptor sites for the most common feelings you've experienced during the last two months. This means that if you've felt the feeling of frustration with your weight every day, then every two months that feeling will get more ingrained in your body. New cells will have the current number of receptor sites and as you continue to feel that feeling every day more receptor sites will be created.

This is why your ego becomes so attached to thinking you are someone who struggles with your weight. The feeling of struggling with your weight gets more and more rooted in every cell of your body every two months.

This is also why, within four to six weeks of January 1st, New Year's resolutions go out the window. The mind is trying to create new feelings, but the cells do not have enough new receptor sites for those feelings to counteract the ones currently in place. Therefore, the *familiar and normal programming* overrides the new behavior.

Chemically and vibrationally, your body is addicted to the feeling of struggling with your weight. Your body has the most receptor sites that not only allow that feeling into your cells but, as a result, create the strongest vibration in your cells. That is why it feels normal for you to struggle with your weight.

If you are not aware this is happening, you have almost **no chance** of success with your weight-loss efforts, and are living in dieting hell! However, now you're learning how your body works, and this book will help you create new receptor sites in your cells for the feelings of peace and love. Yeah!

Memorized Patterns

According to neuroscientist Dr. Joe Dispenza, your memorized patterns created from your subconscious mind run your life ninety to ninety-five percent of the time. That means you are only running your life consciously five to ten percent of your day. The other ninety to ninety-five percent of your day, your emotional addictions are running your life subconsciously through your body![1]

It works like this: When you start feeling differently about yourself, your body will send a signal to your brain to think thoughts that will produce the regular chemical feelings that it's used to. Yes, I said, *"your body will send signals to your brain."* Your body is conscious. Every cell is conscious and the body communicates with the brain all the time.

Do you ever wonder why you think thoughts like, "I'll work out tomorrow" or "I've done so well this week, I will have dessert tonight"? It's because your body actually **sends signals** to your brain to create thoughts that will give it the emotional chemicals it's addicted to. It's like druggies going to their dealer so they can get their fix.

It may be hard to understand that your body sends signals to your brain. I mean, it's supposed to be the other way around, right? Nope.

Your cells are intelligent and they are the mind of your body!

Self-sabotage doesn't happen because you don't have the will-power or self-control to stick with a diet. It happens because

---

[1] Dr. Joe Dispenza, Breaking the Habit of Being Yourself, Hay House, 2012, pp. 62-63

every cell in your body is **familiar with** struggling with your weight and the feelings of disliking your body, and they want to stay that way! It feels normal for you to struggle.

If you were to love your body and be happy with your weight, it **wouldn't feel normal**. It would actually feel wrong. It's a feeling you haven't felt long enough for your cells to be comfortable. You self-sabotage consciously and subconsciously, going back to what feels "normal" in your body.

As if that wasn't bad enough, check this out... Your physical body has memory.

Your body is conditioned to repeat the same behaviors and actions every day. It's like a well-worn path in a forest. If this didn't happen, you would have to re-learn how to walk, tie your shoes, brush your hair and all the other normal activities you do every day.

For example, if you get home and go straight to the kitchen to get something to eat and then sit in front of the TV and eat it, that is a memorized pattern in your body. Your body is conditioned to do it without your conscious thought. The actions of your body walking, opening the fridge, reaching to get a plate and sitting in the same spot on the couch are all *conditioned, memorized patterns.*

It's like driving a car. After you learn how to drive a car, you don't have to think about it. You get in and your body has memorized how to drive and does it without your conscious thought. When you sit in the driver's seat and push the brake, then the gas, then a turn signal, that is your body's memorized conditioned actions, not your conscious thought.

If you went to a different country and drove on the other side of the road, it wouldn't feel right. It would feel uncomfortable and even wrong because your body wants to repeat the same patterns it is used to.

This is, again, why diets don't work. First, when you're about to go on a diet how does it feel? You're not jumping up and down excited to deprive yourself of all the foods you love, are you? You more than likely are feeling a bit excited that *this* time it's going to work and a bit annoyed that you're going on *another diet*! Ugh!

Your body has memorized feelings and behaviors associated with dieting. Even seeing or hearing someone say the word, "Diet" creates a feeling in your body, which is probably the feeling of defeat. This is another reason you should never go on another diet again! Instead of dieting I'm going to teach you an eating plan that leaves you feeling good about yourself and in your body and that you can do for the rest of your life. However, that too isn't going to feel right. It is going to feel different and your job is to give yourself permission to feel different long enough until it feels normal.

Having weight loss goals is another way you sabotage yourself and stay overweight! How do you feel when you have a weight loss goal? Again, not jumping up and down with joy, right? That means your subconscious is set-up to sabotage your efforts every time!

When you're living in a body you love, the feelings will be unfamiliar. It will feel good but it won't feel like you. You must give yourself permission to feel differently and be in the unknown. That is where the magic is.

Here is a practice I give clients in my *Live in a Body You Love* program that will help you understand your emotional conditioning without it being too hard or even related to your weight.

Practice: Permission to Feel Different

Do something different in your day every day for a week, and notice how it feels in your body.

Here are examples:

- *Take a different route to work.*
- *When you first get home, go to the backyard and let the sun shine on your face for two minutes with your eyes closed.*
- *Eat at a new restaurant for lunch or dinner.*
- *Get home and text someone you haven't spoken to in a while and tell them how much you appreciate them.*
- *Brush your teeth using the opposite hand.*

> You get the picture. Notice how different the new pattern feels in your body. Try the new pattern for fourteen days and see how it starts to become a familiar way of being. This is the start to a new memorized pattern.

The new memorized pattern will not be set in your body until your cells divide in two months. This is why you must do new actions and have new thoughts about your weight for at least two-months. We both know that is the challenge. You don't know the new thoughts you will have when you're living in a body you love. Not knowing is a good sign you're about to have a breakthrough.

When I ask a client, "How will that feel?" and they say they don't know, I know we've hit gold! When you don't know how it will feel, that means you're not repeating a past feeling and getting the same result.

You must be willing to feel uncomfortable in the unfamiliar for a while. Don't worry, though. I'm going to give you even more insights and practices to make it easy.

Let's explore the age of your emotional body and let the magic begin!

CHAPTER THREE

The Age of Your Emotional Body

Your biological age and the age of your emotions are two different things. Have you ever seen an adult throw a temper tantrum? I have an example for you.

Client Story

I remember talking with a client and she literally threw a tantrum on the phone. We started talking about her food and she immediately took offense and got angry. I listened as she told me that she couldn't help what she ate and that's just the way it was! It even sounded like she stomped her foot and crossed her arms.

I asked her to tell me the age of the emotions she was feeling. She paused and took a deep breath. I could hear her body relax as she reconnected with me and realized something new about herself. She told me it felt like a five-year-old. I then asked her what happened when she was five years old. She told me that she felt alone and unimportant and her parents would tell her what she could and couldn't eat.

Her five-year-old emotional body was running her behavior as an adult, because she hadn't yet come to terms with her past. There was still anger and pain when she thought of her childhood. We started working on having her accept her childhood without making it wrong or trying to fix anything. Acceptance of all you've been through will heal any emotional trauma.

One reason you are here in a human body is to go through an emotional journey of expansion toward love and forgiveness, and that means growing-up emotionally and transforming past pains. Sweeping painful memories under the rug will only cause emotional triggers and behaviors that will keep you in a body you don't love, forever!

Past hurts and traumas don't have to be big like rape or abuse or neglect, even though they obviously can be. They also can be as simple as something someone said that created an intense negative feeling in your body, and an emotional pattern that doesn't serve you was born.

According to Dr. Joe Dispenza, when you have an intense event happen in your life, it heightens all your physical senses and those signals are sent to your brain. Your brain then releases chemical feelings into the cells of your body and creates an organized pattern that memorizes the situation.[2]

There Is That Word Again: Memorize!

Does a certain song remind you of someone or something? That's because that song was playing when your emotions were heightened. Something or someone caused an intense emotional reaction in your body, and your brain recorded everything about the event. Every time that song plays, your body and brain will bring up the memory and you will relive the emotions of the memorized event.

Regarding low body image and struggling with your weight, an emotionally intense event happened in your past that heightened your senses, and you made an unconscious decision about how you'll keep yourself *safe*. Your brain created the program, or way of being, that became your memorized emotional state, and it still runs your life today.

This means you can be a sixty-year-old woman with a five-year-old emotional body that makes the choices and behaviors in your life. Isn't that crazy? Do you see again why diet and exercise programs will never work? Your adult mind and adult emotions are not running the show. To live in a body

---

[2]   Dr. Joe Dispenza, Breaking the Habit of Being Yourself, Hay House, 2012, pp. 71-72

you love, you must emotionally grow-up and move toward love and forgiveness of yourself and others.

If you don't understand this, you'll keep looking outside yourself for answers. It's only when you understand that you have memorized emotional addictions that come from a younger emotional body that you start to heal them and find peace.

Here is my favorite example…

Are you someone who gets on the scale every day?

What age were you when you first started doing that?

Or what age were you when you first started judging yourself negatively first thing in the morning?

Odds are it was when you were a lot younger.

Client Story

I was coaching a client in her forties who was getting on the scale every day, and was afraid not to get on the scale. She told me that it helps keep her on track and she's afraid that if she doesn't get on the scale she'd balloon up (gain weight).

After asking her the age of her emotional body that wanted to get on the scale, we discovered it was a teenager. I then asked what happened at that age, and she told me that her mother had taken her to a very popular weight-loss program. She had stood there when her mother, who loved her dearly and had the best of intentions, asked the coach what was wrong with her daughter that she couldn't lose weight. She said that she was following the program, but nothing was happening.

Because of this event, my client had memorized the feelings of shame, embarrassment and guilt. She was getting on the scale every day with a teenage emotional body, wanting the scale to tell her that she was good enough and her body was okay. When she realized the truth about the memorized pattern, a feeling of sadness came over her, and we acknowledged and accepted the sadness without making it wrong. It then led to compassion for her teenage self who had to endure that experience.

She had been a slave to the programming of getting on the scale every day of her life and didn't know why she couldn't stop the behavior. When she acknowledged her past emotional trauma without making it right or wrong and had compassion for herself, she was able to put the scale away and start having peace with her body.

Your Emotions Are NOT Who You Are; They Are What You Do.

I will constantly remind you that your emotions are not who you are. They are chemical and vibrational frequencies that are conditioned and memorized in every cell of your body, but they are **NOT who you are.**

Your emotions have a job to do. Their job is whatever you call them. For example, guilt has the job of making you feel guilty. Shame has the job of making you feel ashamed. Your emotions are not **who** you are, they are **what** you feel, which creates how you behave. When you can realize this in the moment that you're having the feeling, it takes back your power and you don't have to behave in a way that matches the feeling.

Think about it like this… a doctor is a person who practices medicine. Practicing medicine is her focus and that creates her actions and behaviors. She chooses to practice medicine and focuses every day on her job, and hence, calls herself a doctor.

Here's how it works when you feel the emotion of frustration with your weight. The "job" of feeling frustrated with your weight is creating actions and behaviors that keep you over-weight because that is what you're focused on. When you sabotage your weight-loss goals, that feeling of frustration with your weight has done its job and you are justified in your behaviors.

Feeling frustrated with your weight is not who you are. It's only a memorized and practiced way of being that coin-cides with calling yourself someone who struggles with your weight. When you understand that who you are and what you feel are two different things, you can notice your feelings without having them affect you or change your behavior.

Your feelings are chemicals and vibrations doing their job in your body because you are paying attention to them. When you pay attention to a feeling, you are feeding it or "paying" it by allowing the chemicals and frequency of that feeling to get stronger in your body. Your behaviors then match your feelings, and that runs your life.

Instead of paying attention to the feeling, explore the age of the feeling and where it came from and have compassion for that version of yourself that created the emotional addiction from that earlier time in your life.

Here is a practice you can do to help you stop paying attention to the feelings that are keeping you overweight and start creating emotional expansion and healing in your body.

Practice: Connecting with the Younger-You

The next time you have a negative feeling, don't make it good, bad, right or wrong. Don't judge the feeling. Simply feel it and FULLY accept it in your body. Let it be okay that it is there without letting it affect your behavior; just notice it.

Here is an example: If you feel sad that you're overweight, put your hand on your heart and say, "Sadness, I know you're here and it's okay. I accept you. You are welcome in my body."

Breathe and FULLY accept the feeling without judging it or making it wrong in any way. Keep accepting the feeling until you feel space between your heart, mind and the emotion. That is starting the disconnect from the emotion running your life. YES!

When you feel space between the feeling and your heart and mind, ask the feeling, "What age are you?" Notice the images or thoughts that come to your mind and watch them like you're watching a movie. Imagine that you're right there with the younger you, watching the event that created the emotional conditioning.

Without trying to fix or judge ANYTHING that happened, tell the younger you they are going to be okay. You know it sucked having to go through that experience and they are going to survive it. Tell them you understand their pain. Then feel compassion for them.

Keep breathing and let yourself feel compassion for the younger part of you that only wanted to feel loved, safe, that they mattered and that everything was okay. That younger part of you was innocent and doing the best they could. They created emotional addictions out of survival. They simply wanted to survive the experience, and they did! It's not their fault the emotional patterns became memorized in your body. They only wanted to get through the experience alive.

Next, find something you can appreciate about them. Appreciation is the first step toward love. It's time to give the younger you the love they wanted and didn't get but so deserved.

This is a daily practice. If this is the only thing you take away from this entire book, it will be enough.

Get a journal and before you go to bed each night, write down three to five things you can appreciate about the younger you. Choose an age that is closest to the time you created emotional patterns that left you struggling with self-love, safety or feelings of worthiness, and move up from there.

Do this for thirty days and watch as you become a happier version of yourself and the weight starts to disappear.

One of the main keys to releasing your emotional addiction to struggling with your weight is to have compassion and appreciation for yourself. It's important, even crucial, NOT to make your feelings, or the situation(s) that created them, wrong.

You can't change the past. Making something you can't change wrong is like trying to move a house with your bare hands. It's futile and you're the only one who gets exhausted, hurt and angry.

The events that happened in your past were experiences that touched your heart and soul, and I believe, were meant to happen for your emotional and spiritual growth.

Don't make ANY part of your life right or wrong. Simply think of it as an experience you had and have compassion for the younger part of you that went through it and created emotional patterns that are still running your life today.

This doesn't belittle what you went through. It brings you peace, and you deserve that! To live in a body you love, start creating a relationship with the younger you based on compassion, acceptance and appreciation.

I've had many clients tell me they don't like the younger version of themselves. Some have told me they even hate them. However, it's not the younger part of them that they hate or are angry at. It's the emotional pattern their younger self unknowingly created in order to survive their childhood.

The younger you may have survived your childhood by being angry, like I was. I was mad all the time, and in a way, the familiarity of that feeling helped me through two divorces, being abandoned, feeling not good enough and more. Like I said earlier, anger ran my life up through my mid-twenties when I lost friends and my twin sister didn't want to be around me anymore. I finally realized I needed to change. It wasn't easy because feeling angry was so normal and familiar to me... and making me miserable.

It's been a long journey toward living in peace, joy and happiness. I can honestly say that's where I am today. I had to make my ego take a chill pill many times when I wanted to be right and tell people how right I was! However, I made a decision a long time ago that connections with others matter more to me than being right. That is how I live my life today. It's not always easy but it's always worth it!

Practice: Give Your Ego a Chill Pill

What is a story you often tell people about who you are regarding your weight?

Remember the woman at the conference who constantly told people about the exercise room she didn't use? What is a story that you tell people when your weight comes up? Is it that you've tried every diet in the world and nothing lasts? Maybe you tell people that you've spent thousands of dollars on trainers and nutritionists and wasted your money.

Whatever the story is, write it down. Write it down completely and then read it to yourself. Then read it out loud in a really loud voice. Read it in a whisper. Read it in a funny voice and then a serious voice.

Notice that it's just a story. You repeat it because you're used to telling it and the way it makes you feel when you tell it is a memorized emotional addiction. It is NOT who you are!

It's merely a story, and guess what? You can share a new story when you are ready to stop being right and instead make peace with your body and experience something new.

If you absolutely feel the need to share your story, change it to "I used to..." Then share your story and be sure to end it with, "and now I..." That will start creating a new feeling in your body that moves you toward a body you love!

The memorized emotions you're addicted to are there because there is a spiritual, physical and emotional expansion needing to happen that will give you relief, freedom and peace in your body. That will begin when you acknowledge your younger self did nothing wrong. They created emotional addictions to survive, which they did! Your job is to stop judging your memorized patterns and past experiences!

If you **take away** the judgment about your life AND acknowledge your feelings, again without making them wrong, they no longer control you. Instead, you'll start to feel a bit of space between your heart and the emotion you're having. That gives you an opportunity to create something new for yourself instead of being a slave to your memorized emotional patterns.

It will take practice because right now you believe that your feelings and behaviors are who you are. They are NOT who you are. They are ONLY who you've memorized yourself to be!

You can change your memorized patterns and you must acknowledge, FULLY accept and create a trusting friendship with your younger-self to shift them. If you stay angry and frustrated at either the event that happened, your younger-self for unknowingly creating emotional addictions or at the memorized patterns themselves, nothing will change and you will remain in dieting hell forever!

Again, you are not a person who struggles with your weight! You are someone who has memorized the emotional patterns, thoughts and behaviors of someone who struggles with their weight.

It's time to explore who you truly are.

Practice: Remember Who You Are

Put your hand on your heart and close your eyes. Feel your heart beating. Ask yourself, "Who is beating my heart?"

Take a deep breath and think, "Who is breathing my lungs?"

Become aware that over 100,000 chemical reactions are happening every second in each of your seventy-trillion cells. Ask, "Who is running my cells?"

When you're in the above exploration, contemplate the following: "If it wasn't possible to feel frustrated that I'm still overweight, or any other negative emotion regarding my weight, what would I feel instead?"

Hmmmmm... really think about that. What would you feel instead if the feelings of frustration, shame, guilt, anger, sadness, hopelessness or any other negative emotion you constantly feel didn't exist on the planet? If they were impossible to feel in your body, what would you feel instead?

You probably don't know because you've experienced the memorized emotional patterns for so long. You may even feel a bit of confusion. Guess what?

That's AWESOME!

If you're in confusion and not knowing, that means you're about to create something new for yourself! When you don't know how you would feel, it's because you haven't experienced it yet and it means you are not experiencing your memorized patterns. YES! Isn't that exciting?

Make it a game! Give yourself FULL permission to REALLY explore what you would feel if you couldn't feel the negative emotions you have every day related to your weight and body image.

What would you feel instead if you couldn't feel the negative emotions you're addicted to?

If you would, please, post what you would feel on my Facebook page. I want to know your answer to that question because it's life-changing and super fun to explore. It also might go into my next book! Go to Facebook.com/WomenBeingFit/

Do this practice after the Connecting with the Younger You practice. They complement each other.

Get ready to be set free from who you think you are and open up to a version of yourself you never knew existed.

In his book *The Untethered Soul,* Michael Singer writes, *"All you have to do is notice who it is that feels the loneliness. The one who notices is already free."* [3]

Substitute any feeling for "loneliness" and you've got it! When you notice yourself noticing who is doing these practices, reading these words, breathing your lungs and beating

[3]   Michael A. Singer, The Untethered Soul, New Harbinger, 2007, p. 86

your heart, you'll realize you are greater than your memo-rized emotions. Now you can start letting the past be what it was without judgment and become a person who lives in a body you love. Yes!

It's going to take practice and you can totally do this! You were born to do this!

CHAPTER FOUR

Three Insights That Bring Your Body Peace

Why do you struggle with your weight and others don't?

Why has this life journey been so hard for you?

Is there a reason for your struggle that you don't know about?

According to Nicolas David Ngan again, in his book *Your Soul Contract Decoded,* before you were born your soul chose your life journey to create the optimal life experience for it to emotionally expand and learn. He writes that your soul chose the time, location of your birth, the culture you were born into, your parents, the entire genetic lineage and more.[4]

---

[4] Nicolas David Ngan, Your Soul Contract Decoded, Watkins 2013, p. 1

I will add that your soul also chose the body you are in as well, because it knew that this body would be the catalyst for the emotional growth it wanted to have. I truly believe it's not a mistake you have the body you have.

Your soul had an agenda for your life and that agenda is conscious awakening to remember who you are, which is love. You are not here to work your tail off for the biggest house and nicest car. You are here to expand your spirit and move toward love and forgiveness of yourself and others through the relationships you have and situations you experience.

You will not be the same person you are right now when you are living in a body you love. You'll be an emotionally and spiritually expanded version of yourself who is happy, feels light and has faith that you can have, do and be anything you want. That is one reason your soul wanted to experience life in a human body.

Your soul knew that challenges, pain and trauma would come into your life. It also knew you would have everything you need to get through them. It would take courage and faith, and your soul was banking on you going through the fire and becoming the phoenix.

It's time to thrive and do what your soul intended to do: expand emotionally and spiritually from your experiences. Are you ready?

Start by looking at your life from a third-person perspective. Think back to all the experiences you've had and everything you've been through. I hinted about this in the last chapter.

My Life in a Nutshell

My parents divorced when I was three and remarried when I was five, and divorced again when I was fifteen.

My first romantic partner cheated and lied to me. My second physically abused me, cheated and stole money from me.

A very close relative committed suicide when I was twenty-one.

In my late thirties, I stayed in the hospital with a dear aunt, who was more like a sister, the last two weeks of her life and watched as she died of cancer.

Then there were the positive things…

I graduated high school mid-term.

I was the first of my family to graduate from college.

I started my own business in my early thirties.

I bought my first home on my own.

I traveled to Scotland, London, Australia, the Bahamas, Alaska, New York and Bali all by myself and had a blast!

I manifested my dream life on the Big Island of Hawaii.

I'm a published author! Yeah!

Each of us has a story. Your story might be similar in some ways and completely different in others. Try this life practice and see how it makes you feel.

Practice: Your Life Movie

The best way to do this practice is to journal about it. Visualization is a good place to start.

Look back at your life as if you are watching a movie and you are the leading character. Think of the main challenges the leading character (you) experienced. Notice how these challenges formed the life of the main character.

Then, think of all the positive events that happened and how those affected the main character.

How do you feel about everything the main character (you) went through? What feelings come up when you look at your life from a third-person perspective?

> Do you feel compassion for the main character in your story?

Every event you've experienced has shaped who you are today but NOT who you will become! That, sweet friend, is up to you.

Compassion is the first step that brings your body peace.

When you feel compassion for everything you've experienced in your life, you will have more peace. Remember, what you went through and your emotional conditioning you created from it, are NOT who you are. When you have compassion for yourself, acknowledge your feelings without making them wrong and start watching when your emotional triggers happen, you can start to shift them and create something new.

Client Story

I had a client who had been struggling with her weight for a long time. We found that when she is overwhelmed and stressed, she goes into *"I don't care"* mode and eats to comfort herself. We named that part of her, *"I don't care."*

We looked back at her life for the first experience that matched that behavior, and found it when she was in her twenties getting her PhD. At the time, she was constantly overwhelmed, alone and frustrated. She started eating to comfort herself.

In her present life, *"I don't care"* shows up when she is stressed out. It's the same feeling she had in her twenties. This emotional addiction literally pulls her to the store to pick up a bag of macaroons and eat the whole bag. It's a familiar feeling and way of being but it's not who she is!

When she finally understood that behavior was an emotional addiction and had compassion for herself for having gone through the first experience that created it, things started to change. She recently texted me, telling me that she went into the store, picked up the bag of macaroons and put it back down! She didn't buy them, which is something she's NEVER done before. Yes! That's what I'm talking about!

You are NOT your emotional addictions. Your habits and ways of being are ONLY memorized patterns created from traumatic experiences. When you really get that, and accept the trauma that happened to you without making it wrong, you will start healing it. You'll then have space to create a new you!

Here is a writing practice that will move you toward more peace in your body.

Practice: Name Your Emotions

Choose a familiar feeling, an emotional conditioning, which triggers a behavior keeping you in a body you don't love. This could be overwhelm, jealousy or not feeling good enough. Then, explore the triggers that create that feeling.

How old does it feel? What triggers the feeling? If it had a name, what would that name be?

Remember, don't make that part of you wrong in any way. In fact, tell that part of you that you FULLY accept it and welcome it into your body. It was created to keep you safe and help you survive the situation that created it.

Tell it you're going to start remembering that you are not your emotional addictions. It was created from a past trauma and you are ready to discover who you are living in a body you love.

Thank your emotional conditioning for wanting to keep you safe and for helping you through the difficult times in your life. The next time that emotional conditioning shows up, say hello to it! For example, *"Hello, 'I don't care.' I know you're here. I fully accept and welcome you right now. It's okay that you're in my body."*

> Don't make it wrong! Your ego's job is to judge. If you stay in judgment, you will keep yourself from the love and peace you desire most. Your practice is to FULLY accept ALL your feelings. Then, have compassion for the younger you having created those emotional addictions.

With awareness, the emotional conditioning that used to cause you to overreact, overeat and do things that don't honor your body, can shift and turn into wisdom.

Here is a quote I will remember for the rest of my life. I learned it from a video I watched with Dr. Joe Dispenza, where he said,

"When you are not emotionally triggered by an intense memory of your past, it becomes wisdom."

The wisdom he is referring to comes when you are triggered to react in a way you've always reacted and you stop yourself and look at the situation in a new way. You then get to choose how you react instead of being a slave to your memorized behaviors.

Surrender and Trust are the second insights that bring your body peace.

Surrender doesn't mean giving up. It means fully accepting the way things are without making them wrong or trying to fix or change them. When you surrender your judgment about your life and your body not being the way you want, and you completely release making yourself wrong for past actions, you bring your body, mind and spirit what you've wanted for so long… peace.

Trusting there is nothing wrong with you and nothing to "fix" creates space between the negative feelings and your heart and mind which bring you peace. When you fight with yourself and make a situation or person (including yourself) wrong, the negative emotional frequency will get stronger in your body and your actions will reflect that feeling. You will forever stay in the fight, and the peace you want can never come to you.

Here is a practice that will help you surrender to your life right now and move you toward peace in your body and with food.

Practice: Surrender to Peace

The morning is the most magical part of your day to practice new feelings. It is also the time your emotional addictions wake up to run your life. When you open your eyes, notice the feeling you have and recognize it as your emotional addiction. Don't make it wrong or try to fix it in any way!

Realize that it's just a feeling. It's not real. You can't see it, touch it, smell it, taste it or hear it. It's only a vibrational frequency in your body. When you truly understand this, the feeling loses its power over you and you can shift it.

To shift the feeling, tell yourself you're ready for peace. You don't want to lose weight or make yourself wrong anymore. You only want peace in your body and peace with food.

Make your intention today that whenever food is around, you're going to choose peace over any other feeling. When you are thinking of food or your next meal, put your hand on your heart and ask yourself, "What is going to give me peace in my body?" Follow your intuition and trust that it will lead you to the peace you're so deserve.

I have all my *Live in a Body You Love* clients say this prayer daily whenever they get stuck and need help.

Live in a Body You Love Daily Prayer:

Guides, Angels, Source of All Things… I know I'm on an emotional healing and awakening journey with my body. Please help me find compassion for all I've been through.

Inspire me to choose foods, thoughts and actions
that nourish my body and soul. Help me live in
peace in a body I love. Thank you, Amen.

This prayer will pull you toward actions and feelings that will leave you feeling good about yourself, and most importantly, having peace in your body. You deserve that! Once you've practiced this long enough, you will naturally move to the real transformation, which is forgiveness of yourself and others.

Forgiveness is the third insight that brings your body peace.

Forgiveness can be hard because it's easier to blame others, including yourself, and be angry for what happened in your life. That will keep you in a body you don't love, forever!

What if your soul knew what was going to happen to you before you were born, and it wanted it to happen?

Have you read the story *"The Little Soul and the Sun"* by Neale Donald Walsch?[5] It's a super cute read.

The story is about a little soul that wants to experience forgiveness. The little soul is talking to another soul about her predicament. The other soul tells her that she'll help her by

---

[5] Neale Donald Walsch, The Little Soul and the Sun, Hampton Roads, 1998.

coming to earth in their next lifetime and doing something horrible to her so she can forgive. The little soul is elated and can't believe the other soul would do that for her. Ha!

The other soul warns her that she'll have to remember who she really is because in order to do this horrible thing, the other soul will have to lower her vibration and forget that she comes from a place of love. The little soul excitedly tells her she won't forget and they both go off to tell God what they've decided.

Even though this story is fiction, it is in line with what Nicolas David Ngan talks about in his book *Your Soul Contract Decoded,* when he writes, "The soul chooses all the primary formative, karmic and ongoing relationships you are to engage in to create the experiences it needs. It contracts with other souls to play specific roles to grow in consciousness."[6]

Think about your life experiences in these terms… what if you planned certain things to happen to you so your soul could emotionally expand and evolve toward a greater level of love for yourself and others? When you give yourself permission to feel that, it releases blame, shame and guilt for past experiences.

Forgiving doesn't say what happened was okay. It says you are no longer going to be a victim. You are letting the anger

---

[6] Nicolas David Ngan, Your Soul Contract Decoded, Watkins 2013, p. 1-2

and hurt release from your body. Haven't you suffered long enough?

Practice: Forgiveness

Think of the worst thing that has happened in your life.

Explore the concept that your higher-self and the higher-self of the other(s) involved chose that to happen to evolve your spirit toward love and forgiveness of yourself and others.

Write down in your journal how you would feel about the experience with this new way of thinking. What changes in your heart? How do you feel about the other soul? How does it change how you feel about yourself and your body?

What new awarenesses come up?

It's not a mistake things happened the way they did. It's all for evolution and movement toward love. I'll explain more later.

When you have compassion for yourself and all you've been through, surrender judgments about how you think things should be and forgive yourself and others, you can start living in a body you love. You may even realize that you no longer want to get on the scale every day and have a machine dictate how you feel about yourself, if that's your normal morning routine.

It's time to have peace. And peace begins in your heart.

CHAPTER FIVE

Food Addiction Starts in Your Heart

I want to introduce you to the most powerful organ in your body... your heart! Your heart is the size of your fist. It was the first organ created when you were conceived.

It generates sixty times more electromagnetic energy than your brain, making it the most powerful organ in your entire body... awesome! Your heart pumps one gallon of blood through your body per minute. It beats 100,000 times a day, about forty-million times a year. There is no machine in history that is more efficient than your heart. Serious amazement happening here!

Check this out... If your heart were severed from your brain, it would still beat. This is because your heart has a brain of its own. The same neurons that fire in your brain are found inside your heart.

Scientists have found 40,000 neurons in the heart that allow it to sense, feel, learn and remember. I LOVE this! As if that wasn't outstanding enough, studies show that the heart may be conscious and connect to a higher intelligence.

A study published in the *Journal of Alternative and Complementary Medicine* found that when test subjects were shown beautiful and horrific images on a screen, their hearts would create a physiological response directly correlating with the upcoming picture **six-seconds** before it was shown.[7] This was even before the brain responded. What? Yep!

Your heart plays a crucial role in your emotional addictions. Remember earlier when I told you that the cells in your body send signals to your brain to think thoughts that create emotions that your body is used to feeling every day?

Those signals start in your heart!

When you had an intense experience that created an emotional addiction, you first felt that feeling in your heart. For example, have you ever had your heart broken?

Yes, most of us have.

---

[7] McCraty, Rollin., Atkinson, Mike., Bradley, Raymond Trevor. (2004). Electrophysiological Evidence of Intuition: Part 2. A System-Wide Process.". [Article] Retrieved from https://www.liebertpub.com/doi/10.1089/107555304323062310

When that happened, your heart felt the pain first. It was like your heart was breaking and it actually was, emotionally. Since it was such an intense feeling, your heart wanted to protect itself from that ever happening again, so it created an emotional wall of protection that Dr. Bradley Nelson, author of *The Emotion Code* calls a "Heart Wall." [8]

Heart walls cannot be seen or physically felt. However, they can, at times, be emotionally felt. You emotionally feel your heart wall when you think of a past experience that was traumatic and you still feel pain. That pain is telling you that you have blocked emotions or a heart wall relating to that experience.

Betrayal Story

I was doing emotion release work on myself around money one day and found a heart wall called "Betrayal." I muscle-tested myself and found that the heart wall was created when I was seventeen years old. What happened to me at that time was that my boyfriend got another girl pregnant and stole $200 out of my bank account to pay for her abortion... Ouch. I actually hadn't thought of that experience in decades.

---

[8] Bradley Nelson, The Emotion Code, Wellness Unmasked, 2011, p. 232

The experience was so intense that my heart created a wall to protect me from being hurt like that again. The cost was that my money was always going up and down and I had trouble finding a loving romantic partner. At one point, I was single for twelve years, and I didn't have a loving relationship that lasted longer than three months until I was in my mid-thirties.

I used to call my sister nearly every day, complaining about how lonely and frustrated I was. You could say I was emotionally addicted to the **feeling of loneliness and frustration** with being single. Those emotions felt very normal to me and I experienced them every day.

I haven't felt like that in years, and even though I'm not currently in a romantic relationship, I feel happy and, more than ever before, I have a sense of peace being single.

Heart walls can create many different feelings in your body, like isolation, depression, not feeling good enough and more! When you have a heart wall, negative emotions will feel more familiar and normal in your body than positive emotions. Heart walls can create what Dr. Nelson calls Addictive Heart Energies (AHE), and this is where it really gets interesting.[9]

AHE are specific frequencies in the heart that can cause addictive behaviors like food obsession. These frequencies

---

[9] Nelson, (2019) Addictive Heart Energy [Article] Retrieved from https://www.healingconsciousness.co.uk/addictive-heart-energy/

and behaviors are not created by the heart, but are created because of heart walls.

Dr. Nelson says, *"Addictive Heart Energy can be thought of as being almost like an intense attractor field in the heart, which is behind the intense pull of addictions. In the same way that the gravitational field of a black hole is so intense not even a beam of light can escape it. An Addictive Heart Energy is, we believe, the driving force behind addictions."*

Your soul came from love and your heart knows this. It needs to feel love, joy and pleasure. It needs these positive feelings so much so that when there is a heart wall created from emotional trauma that is keeping you from love, your heart will reach out and pull you toward things that bring you pleasure, no matter what the cost.

Pleasure, joy and love are the core of who you are and your heart must experience those feelings or it will pull you toward negative addictions like overeating, drugs, sex, alcohol, or any other negative vice to feel pleasure even for a moment. Let me explain this with food addiction…

First, the addiction starts in your heart and most likely is created from an AHE. It feels like a **powerful magnet** has been turned on, pulling you toward food, and there's nothing you can do about it.

Second, the body becomes physically and chemically addicted to the foods you obsess on and habits you create, like eating the same meal in front of the TV or stopping by the same ice cream shop after work every day.

Third, your body and brain become emotionally addicted and conditioned to keeping you overweight and repeating that cycle every day.

After you've done the work in the prior chapters, to end dieting hell, you must start feeling more positive emotions in your heart! Otherwise, your heart will pull you toward negative behaviors that bring it short-term pleasure and long-term pain. If you are someone who hasn't allowed yourself to feel loving, positive thoughts in a long time, this practice will start opening up your heart.

Practice: Let Your Heart Feel Joy

This is another practice that will help you create a better relationship with the younger you AND help you create a heart-based goal!

Write down ten or more things that brought you joy as a kid. What did you love to do?

Here is my list. I loved to…

1. Roller skate
2. Play kick the can

3. Laugh with my sister and friends
4. Play dress-up
5. Walk to my Aunt Terri's who lived three miles away
6. Ride bikes
7. Play on these huge wooden wheels in the backyard
8. Gather chicken eggs at my grandparents' ranch
9. Go swimming at Grandma's pool
10. Pick blackberries by the river

Now it's your turn.

It's probably been a very long time since you remembered some of these things. You may even notice a smile on your face. I did.

Notice the feelings you get as you remember back. If something negative comes up, send it compassion and move to the next fun memory.

Next, think of the last time you really felt joy in your heart and had fun? If it's been a while…

GIVE YOURSELF A BREAK!

Seriously, if you have struggled with your weight most of your life, and haven't been happy or had any fun in a while, give yourself a break! Then, decide right now when you will do something fun and make a plan to do it! Your heart needs you to have fun!

Plan Fun ~ Have Fun ~ Repeat

Have fun at least a few times a month and you'll start to feel lighter in your heart and in your body.

Living in a body you don't love most of your life isn't fun. In fact, is very painful and hurtful to your soul. When you start to give yourself a break and have fun, you'll feel it in your heart. It will feel like a weight has been lifted. When you start feeling emotionally lighter, that is your opportunity to explore and develop self-love. Self-love is crucial if you want to live in a body you love. If you don't love yourself, if you constantly make yourself wrong and put yourself down, you will struggle with your weight for the rest of your life.

"You more than anyone in the entire Universe, deserve your love and affection."— Buddha

Like I've said before, you are on a spiritual journey of emotional expansion that will lead you toward love and forgiveness of yourself and others. Start with becoming awake to your addictive feelings and behaviors. Recognize the age you were when they were created and have compassion for that part of you. Then, start opening your heart and let it love all of YOU!

Your heart came from love. When you keep love from yourself, you go against the energy that created you, and your journey in life will be challenging and, dare I say, miserable. However, when you are willing to start loving yourself, it will change your whole life and bring you more peace and joy than you've ever experienced and you deserve that! It's time to be kind and loving to the one person who truly needs it… YOU!

Your frustration with weight doesn't only come from emotional addictions, but also from a part of you who knows you're meant to love yourself, and you're not doing that. You weren't born to give and give to the people around you and ignore your own desires, needs and wants. Giving yourself permission to have what you want is not selfish! It's actually a loving act that will give you more energy to love and give to others.

Not honoring your desires will leave you resenting others and yourself and feeling frustrated, exhausted and overwhelmed. This is not to say that you should be a narcissist, which I highly doubt you are. There needs to be a balance and what makes you happy MUST be part of that balance.

Practice: Self-Love

There are four actions to create and develop self-love.

Self-Love Action One: Like Yourself

Get in nature and sit on a park bench, large rock or blanket. Nature automatically raises your emotional vibration and relaxes the body. Be somewhere you can watch the clouds. As you sit or lie down, close your eyes and listen to the sounds around you without judgment. Simply notice what's around you in each moment. Feel the wind on your face, arms and torso. Notice the parts of you that are cold, hot or neutral. Recognize that your heart is beating and your lungs are expanding and contracting, all without a to-do list on your part.

Play back the last few days of your life in your mind and ask yourself, *"What is something I like about who I've been in the last few days?"* If something negative comes up, ask yourself, *"What if only the positive things about who I am showed up in my mind right now?"* Let them show up and show you who you are! Allow yourself to see the positive sides of you from the perspective of a third person.

Odds are you don't think the positive things about yourself are very big. Guess what? Those positive things are HUGE! They make you uniquely you. You wouldn't be who you are, making a difference in so many people's lives, without them. It's time to acknowledge ALL the things you like about yourself and write them down. Each night before you go to bed, write at least three to five things you like about yourself.

Self-Love Action Two: Create Balance

To create self-love you need to create balance in your life and in your daily routine. Do you have scheduled downtime to relax, even if it's only for ten minutes?

Do you do things you like doing at least once or twice a month? This is your life and if you're not enjoying it with downtime and fun activities that bring you joy, then you're missing out on experiencing a ton more peace and happiness.

I love this quote from Bob Marley, *"I'm the one who has to die when it's my time to die so I'm going to live my life the way I want to live it."*

He was NOT being selfish by saying this. He was being loving and honoring his unique spirit in the world. When you honor yourself and schedule in rest and fun, you are telling the Universe that you are important and that you matter. Guess what? You do!

Schedule rest and fun into your daily or monthly calendar and watch as you have more confidence and experience more joy.

Self-Love Action Three: Exercise and Food

Exercise and eating food that leaves you feeling good in your body and about yourself are MAJOR acts of self- love. Decide right now that you're going to walk for at least ten minutes after each meal or at least after dinner every night, even if you only walk around your house. Put on some fun music as you walk. It makes walking more enjoyable and music automatically elevates your emotional frequency, making you feel great!

When you're thinking about what to eat, ask yourself this magic question...

What is going to leave me feeling good in my body and about myself?

I'm bringing up this question twice in this book because it is AWESOME and EXTREMELY POWERFUL! If you ask yourself this question and follow your intuition, you're set! It's important to know that what you eat MUST BOTH leave you feeling good in your body AND about yourself. If it's only one of those, don't eat it!

Self-Love Action Four: Create Boundaries and Honor Yourself

Your last act of self-love is to create boundaries and honor who you are in the world. This one will probably be the most challenging, especially if you currently don't honor your boundaries or yourself. Not honoring your boundaries tells the Universe and the people around you that you are not important. Not only will they feel that from you, but you will feel that from you and act accordingly.

If you don't feel important, that feeling was created from a younger version of yourself that experienced an event leaving you not feeling good enough. It's not the truth of who you are. It was only an experience that created a memorized addictive feeling that is running your life today. Do you know what age you were when you first felt unimportant? Can you have compassion for that part of you that had to endure the experience that created that feeling? They deserve your compassion and they deserve you taking a stand for them now at this time in your life, and creating boundaries that honor both the younger part of you and the present you.

Honoring who you are in the world means speaking up. If you have something to say, say it! It's not a mistake that you are in a situation feeling the need to speak. If you don't speak up, you will magnify feeling not good enough and the pattern will repeat itself over and over. The relationships you're in both personally and professionally are not by accident. You're meant to be in those relationships both for your own emotional expansion and theirs. When you are brave enough to speak your truth and honor your opinion, others may not like it, but they will respect you for it and, more importantly, you'll start to respect yourself.

One particular movie speaks volumes about self-love. It's called *"Isn't It Romantic."* If you haven't seen this movie, watch it TONIGHT! I'm not going to tell you much more than that except that it starts with a woman being taken for granted who has no boundaries and isn't speaking up for herself. If that is you, this movie is a MUST SEE!

When you are loving yourself, your heart will feel more joyful and expanded and you'll be able to catch any past emotional addictions and behaviors that take you away from self-love much more quickly. However, be warned! If you are in overwhelm, fatigue or stress mode, your heart will be vulnerable to your emotional addictions and behaviors that keep you in a body you don't love. It's up to you to start creating the life you want and you do that through your heart. You can do this!

A fun way to move toward self-love is to create heart-based goals in regard to your weight. The great thing about heart-based goals is they are a ton more inspiring than creating weight-loss goals, which come from your mind and NEVER last!

Your heart is a hundred times stronger electrically than your brain AND it has a magnetic pull that is five-thousand times stronger than your brain.[10] Have you ever been in love and felt the magnetic pull toward the person you love? The same goes for something you're passionate about. You literally feel drawn to the object of your passion.

That's CRAZY awesome!

Heart-Based Goals

The real reason you want to release weight is not what you think. You may think you want to release weight so you are no longer fat. That goal has never inspired you to release the weight and keep it off for good. Your true reason for wanting to release weight goes much deeper than that. Here are examples of heart-based goals from clients I've worked with.

---

[10] Scott Helton, (2018) Heart Intelligence: The Heart is More Powerful ThantheBrain-GreggBraden&HowardMartin[Article]Retrievedfrom https://cafenamaste.com/heart-intelligence-more-powerful-than-brain-gregg-braden/

I asked clients to finish the following sentence: My heart-based goal is to:

- *Look attractive with my clothes off and the lights on! That will leave me confident, attractive and desirable.*
- *Play hoops with my son. That will let me connect more with him and feel confident and young again.*
- *Hike with my family and be one of the first ones on top of the mountain. That will leave me smiling and feeling that I'm good enough.*
- *Go to my high school reunion close to the size I was when I left! That will leave me feeling confident and good enough.*

Do you see how much more exciting heart-based goals are than "I want to lose weight so I'm not fat"? Your heart-based goal should leave you feeling amazing about yourself and bring you a ton of excitement and joy when you think about it.

Use the next practice to create your heart-based goal.

Practice: Heart-Based Goal

What do you want to experience in your life that being overweight and unhappy in your body are keeping you from experiencing?

On an excitement and happiness scale of one to ten, with one being very boring and ten being elated like you just won the lottery, your desired experience should be a twelve!

Finish these sentences:

My heart-based goal is to…

That will make me feel…

Create at least five heart-based goals. The more the better, but you'll only work with one at a time.

Choose the first heart-based goal that you want to achieve. It should be one that turns your wheels and excites you the most when thinking about it. Be realistic and set a heart- based goal that you can realistically achieve in the next sixty to ninety days. If you set a heart-based goal that is too far in the future, it will not motivate you and may even discourage you. Here are your steps.

Step One: Create a heart-based goal you can achieve in the next sixty to ninety days.

Step Two: Add a date with a reminder alarm in your calendar for when you will achieve your heart-based goal.

Step Four: Do one activity a day that will help you reach your heart-based goal. Each morning ask yourself, "What is one thing I can today to reach my heart-based goal by (goal date)." Then do that as soon as possible.

Step Five: Do your heart-based goal on the goal date and celebrate! (even if it's only you jumping up and down and giving yourself a hug!).

Step Six: Schedule your heart-based goal in your monthly calendar at least once. Don't go more than 60 days without doing your heart-based goal so be sure to add it to your calendar.

Step Seven: Choose your next heart-based goal and repeat these steps.

Heart-based goals are different than weight loss goals because you repeat them every 60 days or more. You don't reach them and never do them again.

Now get excited that these goals are happening in your life sooner than you thought, and let that feeling pull you out of bed tomorrow, perhaps to do your first workout, which can be a simple ten-minute walk. Oh yeah!

I'd love to know a few of your heart-based goals. One might even go in my next book! Please share them with me at https://www.facebook.com/womenbeingfit/

Your next action is to measure yourself.

Notice what you felt when you read that. Did your memorized negative emotions of not feeling good enough or feeling shame surface? I bet something like that did. That's okay, fully accept whatever feelings come without making them wrong. You've gone through the motions of measuring and tracking yourself with diet and exercise programs and it hasn't felt good. However, this is a different way to focus so measuring is also going to be different. I call it, "Get excited to get in your pants!"

Practice: Getting in Your Pants

You're not going to check your weight or write down your inches but you do need to measure yourself to make sure you're moving toward your goal. There is no better way than by the pants you want to fit in! If you have a pair of pants that you consider your "skinny" pants, use those. If you don't, go out and buy a pair of pants one size smaller than you are right now.

Put your pants on the back of the bathroom door. Every morning when you see them, get excited that

---

soon you're going to get in your pants! Let that excitement pull you toward behaviors and thoughts that equal releasing inches.

Make it a game and tell yourself, "I'm getting in my own pants within the next two to three months or sooner!" Say it in a way that makes you laugh.

Laughter is a high vibration emotion in your body that feels great! The more you make yourself laugh about how excited you'll be to get in your own pants, the more you'll be inspired to do things that make it happen!

Test getting in your smaller pants every four to six weeks and feel yourself slowly shrinking into them.

Don't check yourself too often. Checking yourself too often can lead to discouragement that you're not there yet.

This is a journey. Put the days you'll try to get in your pants on your calendar and do not try and get in them before those dates! Measuring every four to six weeks is perfect!

Be sure to mark your calendar to remind yourself to test getting in your pants! Let it excite you and make you laugh.

I know your journey has been painful. What if you didn't take it so seriously? What if you gave yourself a break, had compassion for the younger parts of you that created the emotional addictions you're struggling with and laughed yourself to a smaller you?

Laughter is no joking matter when it comes to your health. The benefits of laughter include:[11]

- Boosting your immune system
- Lowering hormone stress
- Reducing pain and discomfort
- Improving your mood
- Lowering your risk of heart disease
- Improving your resilience
- And more!

You're creating a new way of feeling about yourself, and laughter will be a huge ally on your journey.

After you know your heart-based goal and are working toward getting in your pants, it's time to ask permission from your subconscious and higher-self and see if there is a lesson you haven't learned yet that is keeping the weight on. This is crucial!

---

[11] Lawrence Robinson, Melinda Smith, M.A., and Jeanne Segal, Ph.D. (2018) Laughter is the Best Medicine [Article] Retrieved from https://www.helpguide.org/articles/mental-health/laughter-is-the-best-medicine.htm/

Get Permission and Find the Gifts

Life is about emotional expansion toward love and forgiveness of yourself and others. If you haven't yet learned a lesson around forgiveness and self-love, either the weight will stay on or it won't feel as satisfying as it should feel when you release it, and it will likely come back.

No exercise program, diet or even this book will help you until you allow yourself to move toward self-love and forgiveness, and learning the lessons that created your weight challenges is an ideal way to do that! Find your lesson(s) with this practice:

Practice: Learning Your Lessons

Put your hand on your heart and ask your heart: "What lesson do I need to learn from being overweight and unhappy in my body for so long?" Say to yourself, "I love you... I'm listening." Then, be patient and feel into your heart for the answer(s).

It normally will come up right away. Usually, it's a lesson around forgiveness for yourself or another. It may also be surrendering to things out of your control and trusting that you're taken care of.

If you know what that lesson is, again, feel compassion for the younger part of you that had to experience an event that created the lesson.

Can you open your heart, even a little, to understand that the person(s) who wronged you weren't happy and their souls were facing their own challenges in order to do what they did to you?

Can you give yourself permission to feel compassion for the younger version of them who had to endure an experience they didn't like?

Give yourself permission to see the event from your higher-self's perspective and see that you needed the lesson to move you toward love and forgiveness for yourself and others. Be kind and patient with yourself.

You may have to forgive over and over until you feel the shift. The last chapter on Ho'oponopono will give you a practice you can do every day that leaves you with peace, love and forgiveness for yourself and others. For now, realize there is a lesson your weight is holding for you. It's your job to experience the lesson and move toward love and forgiveness. You can do this!

The lessons in your life always move you toward love and forgiveness. They are part of the evolution of your soul and that is one reason you're in a human body.

Find the Gifts

Events happen to give you the gift of yourself. You wouldn't be who you are today if you didn't go through what you went through. Even if an event was really painful, it has given you part of your personality. For example, if you experienced sexual abuse, you can have compassion and understanding for others who've experienced the same. You may even be able to help others through it. That is the gift. Can you find the gifts in your life experiences that were painful but created something positive in your life?

When you look at your life as a set of events without making them wrong, but instead see them as opportunities that move you toward self-love and forgiveness, you gain what you really want, which is peace. When you have peace in your body, your weight will no longer be an issue and it will melt away.

After you have learned the lesson(s) and found any gifts that your weight is here to give you, you must tell your subconscious mind what your heart-based goals are by speaking its language. That will put your subconscious and conscious minds on the same page. Oh yeah!

The Language of Your Subconscious Mind

Your subconscious mind doesn't speak in words. This is why positive affirmations often don't work! Speaking words to your subconscious mind sounds like Charlie Brown adults, "Wah, Wah, Wah." It doesn't get it. The language of your subconscious is your five senses: taste, smell, touch (feeling), sight and sound.

The most powerful senses that communicate the best with your subconscious are touch (feeling), sight and sound. When exploring your heart-based goals through these three senses, your subconscious and conscious minds can get on the same page!

Before you communicate with your subconscious mind, it's important to get in a full brain posture and fire up both the right and left hemispheres of your brain so your entire body gets the messages. Your right and left brain are responsible for different parts of your experiences. The left brain focuses on language, logic and numbers, while the right brain focuses on emotions, expression and imagination. When you have an experience that creates an emotional addiction, these memories are stored in either the right or left hemisphere of your brain.

When doing healing practices like the one I'm going to share with you, you can optimize your results by turning on both sides of your brain as you do the practice. The easiest way to do this is by crossing both your arms and legs. Science has shown that when your arms, legs, ankles or hands cross your midline, it fires up the opposite side of your brain even if you're focused on something that doesn't involve that side of the brain. Amazing!

You can do this simply by crossing your legs or ankles, crossing your arms, and if you're really talented, cross your wrists and interlace your fingers. Now you're in a whole brain posture firing up both the right and left hemispheres of your brain.

Get into a whole-brain posture and do the following practice.

Practice: Speak the Language of Your Subconscious

As you are in a whole-brain posture, see yourself experiencing your first heart-based goal. Put it in the first-person, present-tense like it is happening now.

Communicate with your subconscious by answering these questions:

- Where in your body do you feel the experience of achieving your first heart-based goal?

- What do you hear people saying about you now that you've reached this goal?
- What are you saying to yourself?
- What do you see yourself doing?
- What do you see other people doing around you because you've reached this goal?
- How does that make you feel?

Explore each of these inquiries with each of your heart- based goals until you can see, hear, and feel them in your entire body.

Take your time and let your subconscious understand your heart-based goals.

When you're complete, lock in the experience by uncrossing your legs, putting them on the floor and touching your fingertips together: thumb to thumb, first finger to first finger and so on. Then, keeping your chin up, look at the ground. Sit like that for at least ten-seconds to ground the experiences in your body.

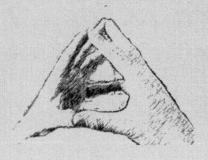

> Add this practice to your daily routine and do it for two minutes in the morning and two minutes in the evening for thirty days. Mark it on your calendar and watch what happens.

If you create heart-based goals and don't line up your sub-conscious mind, then you are ninety to ninety-five percent certain to fail! Your subconscious needs to get the picture in a language it understands. Otherwise, it will stay with the programming it is running.

Remember, your body will want to stay in its emotional addiction of self-loathing. That feels normal. It's best to do this practice first thing in the morning before your brain and body have time to wake up. You can do it before you get out of bed or before you go to sleep. You also don't have to be sitting. You can do this lying in your bed.

I learned part of this technique when I became certified in Psych-K. Psych-K is a method of creating lasting change in your life so you can move toward what you want.

In my *Live in a Body You Love* program, I personally take participants through this practice when they come to the retreat on the Big Island of Hawaii. Maybe one day I'll get to meet you here! Another method of change you will do if you join me in Hawaii is mirror practices.

Mirror Practices

Doing mirror practices is crazy powerful work on your subconscious mind! You currently have a relationship with the image you see in the mirror. That relationship is keeping you at your current weight and fitness level.

In order to have peace and live in a body you love, you must create a new relationship with your image in the mirror. This means, you guessed it… looking at your reflection. When you look at yourself and you don't like what you see, you are sending a powerful message to your subconscious mind that says, "Keep inspiring me to do things so I don't like my body."

Your subconscious only understands what it feels, sees and hears. If you look at your reflection and get an intense feeling of loathing, that message will create more experiences like that.

Being brave enough to do mirror practices will be a complete game changer in your life. It's going to take time and I know you can do this! Give this practice a try.

Practice: Mirror Practices

In the morning after you've gotten ready and before you leave the bathroom, say to yourself, "I'm curious what it will feel like to look at myself in the mirror and feel confident knowing I look amazing!"

Then look at yourself in the mirror and notice what comes up for you. If anything negative comes up, don't make it wrong! Completely accept it and tell yourself it's okay to feel this way. Don't stay in that feeling for more than a few seconds. Ten-seconds is too long.

Look away from the mirror and give yourself compassion for creating the negative feeling that came up. Then, take a deep breath and practice it again… "I'm curious what it will feel like to look at myself in the mirror and feel confident knowing I look amazing!"

Look at yourself again in the mirror. Explore what it will feel like standing there feeling confident. Play the game and see if you can experience the feeling. Keep repeating this process until you feel an emotional shift that gives you a peek at how amazing and confident you are!

One day, sooner than you think, you'll look in the mirror and feel confident knowing you look amazing!

Congratulate yourself for trying something new and tell yourself, "I'll see you tomorrow, beautiful!" As you leave the bathroom, think of things you are grateful for and smile as you think of them.

Add this practice to your daily routine for thirty days and see what happens. Oh yeah!

There will be times when you don't want to look in the mirror and do this work. At those times, have compassion for yourself. Don't make yourself wrong for not wanting to look at your image. Simply tell yourself that you accept that feeling. Welcome it in your body. It's okay that it's there. Then ask, "Who is feeling this feeling? What age is this emotional body?"

Have compassion for that younger part of you. It's been painful to look in the mirror and accept the image staring back at you. The image you created up until now was created from traumatic experiences where you didn't feel good enough, lovable or worthy. The younger you who created your current image was in a lot of emotional pain. Show them compassion for what they went through. It's time for them to live in peace and only you can give that to them by doing this work in a loving and fun way.

Remember, finding ways for your heart to feel pleasure will pull you toward reaching your goals! It's time to put yourself first and enjoy your life!

Life is only a game. It's a game of emotional expansion or staying stuck and making yourself a victim. It's your choice! There is no right or wrong. There are only experiences. I want to free you from an experience you NEVER have to do again!

Never Try to Lose Weight!

When you try to lose weight, you are compromising your heart-based goals and disrespecting yourself. Trying to lose weight tells your subconscious that you think something is wrong with you. There is nothing wrong with you! There is nothing to fix!

You are addicted to memorized patterns that your subconscious created to help you survive an unpleasant experience. That doesn't mean something is wrong with you. It means you're a human being doing the best you can with the cards life dealt you! Give yourself a break and have compassion for all you've been through. The feelings you experience when you try to lose weight bring up your memorized behaviors of not feeling good enough and you set yourself up for sabotage and failure!

Your new goal must come from your heart and lead you toward self-love. When you focus on self-love and confidence, the weight will release from your body and it will stay off! Do this practice for no less than a month!

Practice: New Self-Love Behavior

Keep a notepad with you for two to three days. Make three columns: Away from Self-Love, Emotional Age, New Self-Love Behavior.

In column one, write down all the things you do that take you away from loving yourself. You can even name them to help you remember what they are.

In the second column, write down the emotional age of that behavior and see it as a memorized pattern in your body. When you write the age, see the younger-you who created the behavior out of survival, and have compassion for them.

In the third column, write your new self-love behavior. This new behavior must come from your heart. It needs to leave you feeling good about yourself and in your body. That is crucial!

Next, tell your subconscious what your new self-love behavior is by using the Speak Your Subconscious Language practice you read about earlier. Remember to sit or lay-down and cross your arms and legs comfortably.

See yourself doing your new self-love behavior.

- What will you hear people saying to you?
- What will you be saying to yourself?
- How will you feel in your body?
- Where will you feel that feeling in your body?
- What will you be seeing yourself do and how will that feel?

Take your time and really get this in your body. Lastly, use the mirror practice to anchor your new self-love behavior. Look in the mirror as if you've been practicing your new self-love behavior for the past year.

Feel proud and confident. Get curious to see what shows up for you out of this practice. It's going to be new, unknown and awesome! Yes!

Your self-love action might be something you've never done before that you've always wanted to do, like taking a painting class or joining a singing group. This is where you start to awaken to who you truly are. When your actions and behaviors are more loving, fun and pleasurable, you'll easily move toward a body you love and the weight will be a thing of the past.

Discover what brings you joy! It's not going to look like anything you've ever experienced. Remember, if you know what it's going to look like, it will give you the same results you've always gotten.

Self-love behaviors are new and you will not know the outcome. You may even feel a bit insecure because you've never done it before. Be willing to feel uncomfortable so you can feel the pleasure of moving toward a body you love. You deserve that! When you know your new self-love behavior, repeat it often. Consistency is the key to change. Get your body used to the new behavior so it can let go of the old one and feel peace.

It will take time and you can do this! You're meant to do it! It's time to claim the life you want to have, and self-love is the path to get you there!

CHAPTER SIX

Boost Your Weight Loss

To end dieting hell, think about creating a new food plan versus going on another diet. When you go on a diet, you immediately have conditioned feelings and beliefs about deprivation and disliking the experience. That is a HUGE reason you fail! Start thinking of your food in terms of creating a new eating plan that leaves you feeling good in your body and about yourself, and you'll create peace with food in no time!

In this chapter, you will learn the best insights from my *Boost Your Weight Loss* six-week detox program.

Does this sound like you? You…

- Crave either sugar or salty foods.
- Feel stressed if you think about cutting out these foods.
- Have withdrawal symptoms when you stop eating them.

If so, you are probably addicted to those foods but it's not the way you think.

Here is an important piece of information… food manufacturers have designed foods knowing the exact amount of salt, sugar and fat that trigger the addiction center in your brain. This means these foods will create chemicals in your body and brain that no amount of willpower can overcome! This should be criminal and they can legally create food that has this kind of power over you! This is why it is so hard to stop at one brownie, one potato chip or one cookie. Most processed foods and nearly ALL store-bought baked goods, pastries, candies, chips, muffins, sodas and more are scientifically created to hit the bliss factor in your brain that triggers eating addiction. It's an addiction that is stronger than cocaine.

If you eat food designed to create an addiction, you will overeat, no matter how much you say, "I'm only going to have one." Willpower is null and void when it comes to the chemicals in your brain and body created from these types of foods. Seriously, someone should be going to jail for this. It's like a drug dealer spiking the water in a school so kids are hooked on a drug they didn't know they were being exposed to. If that were to happen, someone WOULD be going to jail! Not in the food industry. They have FULL permission to spike your punch without you being aware of it and they don't have to tell you a thing!

Here's an example of what I'm talking about. One type of sugar, when consumed, turns off the hormone leptin. Leptin is responsible for telling your brain that you're no longer hungry. If this hormone is turned off, you will keep eating or drinking without a clue that your body is full. This so-called food is high fructose corn syrup (HFCS).

HFCS is in nearly all sauces, baked goods, candies, sodas and more! It's cheaper than regular sugar, it's sweeter and creates a chemical addiction in your brain. This is why you can drink a thirty-two-ounce soda in less than an hour, no problem, but not thirty-two ounces of water in an hour. The water allows the signal in your brain to clue you in that you're full, but the HFCS ingredient in the soda turns that signal off, so you keep drinking.

The worst part is that food manufacturers have you addicted to the deadliest drug on the planet: SUGAR! Sugar addiction is stronger than heroin addiction.

Doctor Mark Hyman hit a home run when he said, *"The $1-trillion industrial food system is the biggest drug dealer around, responsible for contributing to tens of millions of deaths every year and siphoning trillions of dollars from our global economy through the loss of human and natural capital."*[12]

Sugar affects nearly all your organs and systems in a negative way, from reducing the elasticity in your skin causing wrinkles, negatively affecting your eye-sight, feeding your bad gut bacteria, which makes it nearly impossible to lose belly fat to

---

[12] *Fed Up*. Dir. Stephanie Soechtig. 2014. Film

being one of the main food sources for cancer! Cancer has insulin receptors, so it loves sugar! The bad bacteria in your gut that contributes to your weight not budging also loves sugar.

Your gut health is one of the four most important keys to release inches and move your body toward health. The other three are insulin, toxins and hormones. I don't specialize in hormones, but my colleagues and dear friends Dr. Ritamarie Loscalzo and Dr. Lindsey Berkson do. They are both nutritionists, international speakers and authors. For more information about hormones, please look them up online!

Let me tell you about the number-one body system that can release weight quickly and safely when it's running optimally. It's your gastrointestinal tract, better known as your gut! Gut health is crucial to releasing inches. I mean Numero UNO!

Here is a short list of what your gut does for you...

- Breaks down food so nutrients can be absorbed.
- Regulates your hormones.
- Is home to eighty percent of your immune system.
- Plays a major role in clean, healthy skin.
- Makes ninety-five percent of your serotonin — the happy feelings!

Many studies now show that most diseases start in your gut. Maintaining a healthy gut is not only important for weight loss, but for optimal health as well!

One of the first actions I have my clients take is to start consuming a high-quality probiotic with at least sixty-billion CFUs to support their gut health. The one I recommend is by Physician's Choice and you can get it on Amazon. When you take a probiotic, it literally creates colonies of good bacteria in your gut. That is what CFUs stand for: "Colony Forming Units." When your gut is back in balance, your sugar cravings will be a thing of the past!

Note: If you are taking medications, you'll want to wait and take your probiotic 3-hours before or after your meds to make sure they are absorbed in your body.

For added support, you want your probiotic to have prebiotics in it. Prebiotics feed your good gut bacteria. Now you have new colonies of bacteria in your gut and you're feeding them to keep them nice and happy! YES!

If you're addicted to sugar, rarely eating leafy greens or vegetables and not drinking enough clean, filtered water, chances are you have symptoms that your gut needs a detox.

Here are six signs your gut could use a detox:

You…

1. Have trouble eliminating solid waste at least two times a day.
2. Lack energy
3. Struggle with mental focus.

4. Have weight that won't budge especially around your belly.
5. Feel gassy and bloated after meals.
6. Have bad breath.

If any of those sound like you, it's probably time for a detox. You can discover if your body needs a detox by taking my **free** quiz at: www.WomenBeingFit.com/DetoxQuiz

Have you ever seen a man who looks pregnant? As much as he'd like to think that's muscle in his gut, it is far from that! He has been eating poorly for so long that his gut is showing the effects of it. His gut, more than likely, has undigested fecal matter and toxins stored in his fat. Yes, I said undigested fecal matter.

It works like this… your body has amazing backup plans to keep you safe! When your liver, the main organ that detoxes your body, is overloaded with sugar, medications or other toxins, your body will wrap fat around excess toxins to keep them away from vital organs, and then stores it on your belly!

This is a HUGE reason to do a detox! Not only will it release toxins out of your system, but it will get things moving optimally through your gut again, leaving you feeling a TON better! You should always check with your doctor before doing a detox or adding supplements to your program.

If you want to release inches naturally, get off sugar, take a probiotic, cleanse your liver and colon, and you'll see results almost instantly!

Next, start drinking half your body weight in ounces of filtered water, not tap water, a day. Someone should be going to jail for tap water, too! What they allow in our tap water is criminal!

An article in *Women's Health* magazine showed the following:

- In 2015, seventy-seven million Americans lived in areas where their tap water systems were in violation of safety regulations.
- In 2016, thirty-three states had drinking water that contained unsafe levels of PFAS, a class of industrial chemicals linked to cancer, hormone disruptions and high cholesterol.
- In 2011, the federal government spent $11 per person on pipes, pumps and water plants compared to $76 per person in 1977, thirty-four years prior!

Bottom line…

Don't Drink Tap Water!

I don't cook with it or give it to my dogs! Find a good water filter that filters chlorine, fluoride, lead, mercury and other toxins. Buy a stainless steel water bottle, not aluminum or plastic, and drink only filtered, purified water daily. You want to drink half your body weight in ounces of water a day to optimally hydrate your body.

To find the best water filters, visit https://healthykitchen101. com and put "water filter" in the search box. A list of the best water filters for the current year will come up. Order one on Amazon.

I also use a shower filter because your skin is the largest organ of your body, and when it heats up from hot water, it more easily takes in chemicals that are in the water.

Hydrating is crucial not only for health, but for releasing inches! A twelve-week study showed that participants who drank seventeen ounces of water before each meal lost 4.4 pounds more than those who did not.[13] Yeah! Research also shows that the more water you drink, the better! For every additional eight ounces of water you consume, it speeds up your metabolism by as much as twenty-four calories a day, which is potentially 8,760 calories a year. Awesome!

Another huge support to gut health is taking a digestive enzyme with most meals. It supports your stomach's ability to breakdown food so nutrients are better absorbed and your meal moves to the next part of digestion easily, leaving you feeling energized. If you feel bloated after meals not only is

---

[13] by Adda Bjarnadottir, MS, (2017), How Drinking More Water Can Help You Lose Weight [Article] Retrieved from: https://www.health-line.com/nutrition/drinking-water-helps-with-weight-loss#section1

it hinder your weight loss but you could end up with acid reflux or other digestive issues. Digestive enzymes make a big difference.

If you are prone to acid reflux, it isn't because you have too much acid in your stomach, it's because you don't have enough. This is why you'll see people popping Tums tablets like it's candy. That is not helping you. That person is doing the exact opposite of what their body needs. Taking a digestive enzyme would be a much better choice to relieve their acid reflux and move them toward better health.

After you've cleansed your liver and colon and are supporting your gut with good probiotics and digestive enzymes, your next step is looking at your food choices.

Here is the magic question again that I told you about earlier…

What can I eat that will leave me feeling
good in my body and about myself?

This question will support you to make food choices that honor living in a body you love! Remember there will be times when you're stressed-out and tired. At those times, it's VERY easy to go back to your memorized emotional patterns and making choices that don't serve you. Here's a practice that will help put you back on track…

Practice: Shake It Out

If you are feeling tired, stressed, anxious, frustrated, angry or any other negative emotion, and you have a meal coming up, shake your body for thirty to sixty-seconds.

I mean shake, shake, shake every inch of your body! Shake your legs like there is a dog biting your shoe, your arms like there are a ton of bees swarming you, and your hips like you've signed up for a fast and furious hula class. Shake every inch of you for thirty to sixty-seconds, nonstop!

When you shake your body, you create a state-change and it automatically increases energy and shifts your emotions. When you're done, notice how much better you feel in your body. You will have more energy and feel a tingling sensation throughout your whole body. Oh yeah!

Now you can ask the magic question:

What can I eat that will leave me feeling good in my body and about myself?

Put your hands on your heart and tell yourself, "I love you. I'm listening."

Listen to your heart and trust what comes up.

Track Your Meals:

You can also make it a game and track your meals on a calendar! Decide how many meals in a month you want to finish feeling good in your body and about yourself. Mark it on a calendar. Here is an example: Let's say you want to complete sixty meals that leave you feeling good about yourself and in your body.

There are ninety meals in a month, so that's a little over half. Put "60" at the top of your calendar. Every time you finish a meal feeling good about yourself and in your body, put one line on that calendar day. At the end of the month, add up the lines to see if you met your goal.

For the next month, see if you can meet or beat your goal last month. YES!

This will take practice because you're not used to it. Getting started is fairly easy. Remember, around the fourth to sixth week, your body will want to go back to what feels normal. This is the time to get support. Ask a friend to help you stay on track. Join my online *Be Fit* workout program or do something that supports you to keep going. I HIGHLY recommend that you put a reminder on your calendar around week five to get more support! It will happen like that every four to six weeks for a while. Keep finding support at that time and you'll see amazing progress!

The great thing is that when your body is detoxed, your liver and colon are running optimally, and you've released your emotional addiction to the struggle to lose weight, you will be empowered to eat in a way that leaves you feeling good about yourself. That will be a game changer for your life! You can do this!

Now it's time to understand the food you eat. I'm going to share a completely new way of understanding food that I found from an amazing scientist and an incredible doctor. When you start eating this way, not only will inches melt off your body, you'll have more energy, better sleep, better mental clarity, more self-confidence and more! Yeah!

Understanding Food

I suggest you order the book by Raymond Francis called *Never Be Sick Again*. Throughout his book, he says, "A diet that focuses on anything other than meeting the nutritional needs of cells allows your body to get sick."[14]

Food is information! It tells your body so many things, like how to control your metabolism, appetite, immune system,

---

[14] Raymond Francis, M.Sc., *Never Be Sick Again*, Health Communications Inc. 2002, p.89

energy, hormones, memory, how to hold onto fat or release fat, and more! The foods you eat, water you drink, substances you put on your skin (lotion, soap, cleansers), exercise you do, and levels of stress you have in your body are all factors that move you toward health or disease!

For optimal health and weight loss, you must understand three main food categories:

- Good fat
- Clean protein
- Unrefined carbohydrates

Even though all of these foods are important, if I was going to prioritize them, I would put good fat first!

Good Fat

Good fat is a macronutrient, which means your body requires it in large amounts for optimal nutrition. Good fat is found in whole, live foods, not processed foods.

Here is why I would put good fat as number-one: It is absolutely essential to the over seventy-trillion cells of your body because it makes up your cell membrane (outer layer). Your cell membrane does two things: It regulates what goes in and out of your cells and it stores electricity. If your cells' membranes are not strong because they don't have the right **quality** of fat to support them, they will leak out vital nutrients, allow toxins in and not maintain optimal energy. This will affect your health and cellular communication, especially in your brain.

Bad fats, like those found in processed foods, fried foods and baked goods, reduce your energy, cause inflammation, hormonal imbalances, fat storage, mental clarity issues and more!

The good fat your cells need is called essential fatty acids (EFAs). Your body needs a near equal 1:1 ratio of EFAs coming from omega-6 and omega-3. Most Americans consume too much omega-6 and very little omega-3.

Like I said earlier, food is information. When you eat good fat, you're telling your body to...

- Support your hormones
- Support your brain function
- Feel satisfied with your meal
- Support your energy system
- Release weight
- Improve your nails and hair
- Help vitamin absorption
- Decrease inflammation
- Look younger
- Sleep better

Can you see how important eating good fat is for your health?

One thing many clients believe is that eating healthy isn't going to taste good. However, eating good fat is designed to satisfy your hunger. Isn't that wonderful? Something that is crucial for your body is also going to leave you feeling content with your meal. Super awesome!

Here are sources of good fat:

- Avocados
- Nuts and seeds
- Olives
- Coconut oil (cook with this or ghee)
- Olive oil (use ONLY on salads, not to cook with, unless it is formulated for high heat)
- Wild-caught fatty fish
- Barlean's flax oil
- Udo's Choice Perfected Oil Blend

As important as it is to know what good fat is, it's just as important to be aware of bad fat.

Here are sources of bad fat that you want to reduce or eliminate from your diet. (Every cell win your body depends on it.):

- Canola oil
- Corn oil
- Cottonseed oil
- Peanut oil
- Safflower oil
- Soybean oil
- Sunflower oil
- hydrogenated oils

When you eat foods containing these oils your cells use it to build their membranes. They then end up with thin, outer walls that are fragile versus more elastic like a balloon. That compromises the cells' ability to absorb vital nutrients it needs and keep toxins out. You want your cells membrane to be made up of healthy fats, not fats which make you vulnerable to disease.

You may be saying, "But Michelle, most of the store-bought foods I buy, like my chips and cookies, all have these bad oils. What should I do?"

Believe me, I get it. I love my organic tortilla chips and they have canola oil in them so I no longer buy them. Now I make my own potato chips. I bake sweet potatoes in coconut oil nearly every Sunday night and have them for the entire week.

Guess what? You can have your favorite foods! You'll only need to make them yourself. You know that beautiful stove you have, use it! Yes, this will take time and your health is worth it! You'll have more energy, better clarity and memory and start to see inches release from you body.

"To keep the body in good health is a duty... otherwise we shall not be able to keep our mind strong and clear." —Buddha

If you are truly ready to end dieting hell, you must take seriously what you put in your body and the best way to do that is to cook for yourself or order food you know is prepared without harmful substances. There are chefs around the world, maybe even in your local area, who prepare healthy meals you can pick-up or have it delivered to your door. One such chef is Beth Freewomon, founder of IAmTheOpenHearth. com a company based in Santa Cruz, California. There she makes amazing gluten-free, organic, plant-based meals that her clients order weekly. The food is incredible. If you don't have time to cook healthy meals for yourself, find a company that can do it for you. You deserve that!

Cooking Oil Warning

According to Raymond Francis in his most awesome book, *Never Be Sick Again*, he states that most supermarket oils heated above 392 degrees Fahrenheit, will change the molecules turning them into trans-fats, which are harmful to your body.[15] The best oil to cook with is coconut or ghee, which is clarified butter from grass-fed, pasture-raised cows.

How much good fat should you eat per day? The amount of fat you need is based on the **calories** your body needs and the diet you choose.

For a Mediterranean diet, where you consume mostly plant-based foods, vegetables, legumes, minimal fish and other

---

[15] Raymond Francis, M.Sc., Never Be Sick Again, Health Communications Inc. 2002, p.97

meats, you'll need **thirty-five to forty percent of your food from good fat.**[16]

Here are the recommended amounts in grams and table-spoons (tbsp):

- 1,500 calories (small-frame person): About 58–67 grams of fat per day or 19–22 grams per meal (1.5 tbsp).
- 2,000 calories (medium-frame person): About 78–89 grams of fat per day or 26–30 grams per meal (2 tbsp).
- 2,500 calories (large-frame person): About 97–111 grams of fat per day or 32–37 grams per meal (2.5 tbsp).

Start consuming good, healthy fat with most of your meals and give your cells the support they need to keep you healthy as you release inches and feel great in you body! Yes!

Clean Protein

The next food I would put on the priority list would be clean protein, either from plants or grass-fed, pasture-raised meats with no hormones or antibiotics added. Protein is also essential for your body. It builds, maintains and repairs nearly

---

[16] Franziska Spritzler, RD, CDE (2016). Fat Grams – How Much Fat Should You Eat Per Day?[Article] Retrieved from https://www.health-line.com/nutrition/how-much-fat-to-eat

all the tissues in your body, including your bones, muscles, blood, hair, nails and organs.

When you eat clean protein, you are telling your body to repair and build your tissue, increase muscle mass, strengthen and maintain bone mass, boost your metabolism, increase your body's ability to burn fat and more!

Good sources of clean protein include:

- Quinoa (favorite)
- Eggs
- Nuts and seeds
- Hemp, flax and chia seeds
- Chickpeas (hummus)
- Spirulina
- Lentils
- Wild-caught fish (limit to once a week)
- Cage-free, hormone and antibiotic free chicken

I didn't include beef on the list because I feel eating it is not healthy and contributes to many diseases. Beef is one of the first foods doctors tell you to decrease in your diet if you have heart disease. Plus, conventional farming is inhumane and contributes to a host of global issues.

Buying meat, eggs or dairy from conventional farms that do not say organic, pasture-raised, hormone-free or antibiotic-free, you are putting toxins in your body and contributing to the pollution in the world and the torture of animals.

Factory farms cause thirty-seven percent of methane (CH4) emissions, which has more than twenty times the global warming potential of CO2 (carbon dioxide). Shockingly, approximately 1,800 gallons of water are used per pound of beef produced in America.

If you want to help conserve water and clean up the Earth, the best thing you can do is to not eat meat or only buy it from farms you know practice conservation, pasture-raising and do not use hormones or antibiotics.

My last statement on factory farming is that animals in those environments die a terrifying and painful death. The hormones secreted at that time go into their tissues, which is turned into meat that is sold in stores. When you consume that quality of meat, it affects your energy and emotions. If you are going to purchase meat, dairy and eggs, my highest recommendation is to purchase food from organic farms that have humane practices. Conventional factory farming is one of the most horrendous industries allowed to produce food for human consumption in the world!

My dream is that someday soon we will live in a world where all sentient beings feel safe and are treated kindly.

These three quotes say it all:

"People eat meat and think they will become as strong as an ox, forgetting that the ox eats grass." — Pino Caruso

"Nothing will benefit human health and increase chances for survival of life on Earth as much as the evolution to a vegetarian diet." — Albert Einstein

"If slaughterhouses had glass walls, we'd all be vegetarian." — Paul McCartney

In the official journal of Kaiser Permanente, physicians are told that healthy eating may best be achieved with a plant-based diet, and limited meats, dairy and eggs as well as all refined and processed foods.[17]

If your goal is to be healthy, have great energy and feel good in your body, you'll want to lean toward plant-based diets. Dr. Neal Barnard, President of the Physicians Committee for Responsible Medicine, had this to say about plant-based diets, "Plant-based diets are the nutritional equivalent of quitting smoking."[18]

To really understand how to eat a more plant-based diet, check out my friend and colleague Ocean Robbins and his new book, *31-Day Food Revolution: Heal Your Body, Feel*

---

[17] Michael Greger, M.D. (2016). Nation's Largest Health Care Organization Wants to Make Plant-Based Diets the New Normal. [Article] Retrieved from https://foodrevolution.org/blog/food-and-health/plant-based- diets-the-new-normal/

[18] Michael Greger M.D. FACLM, (2017) Plant-Based Diets as the Nutritional Equivalent of Quitting Smoking. [Article] Retrieved from https://nutritionfacts.org/2017/08/01/plant-based-diets-as-the-nutritional-equivalent-of-quitting-smoking/

Great and Transform Your World. It will change your life for the better! Oh yeah!

Another important fact worth mentioning is if you value eating non-GMO (Genetically Modified Organisms) foods, do not consume meats from conventional factory farms. Conventional factory farms feed their animals GMO corn, soy and alfalfa. If you are eating meats from conventional factory farms, you're consuming GMOs! One of the first things GMO foods were designed to do is be resistant to weed killers and pesticides. If you are eating food that is resistant to substances that kill weeds and insects, what do you think it's going to do in your body?

When GMO companies say that GMOs are safe, their logic baffles me, but money can buy any research results they want. Ugh!

The dairy industry is another industry you need to be VERY aware of! First, dairy should never have been on our food pyramid. Lobbyists basically bought their spot there! Watch this video called Dairy Doubts by Dr. Michael Klaper. Find it on YouTube at **TinyUrl.com/DairyDoubts.** This video is amazing and shows you just what the dairy industry is all about.

Here is some truth about dairy you should know. Your body becomes more acid when metabolizing dairy, so instead of building your bones and tissues, it pulls calcium from them. Most of the population is allergic to dairy, causing inflammation in the body when they consume it. (It's been shown that fifty percent of all children are allergic to dairy.)

Here are three reasons not to consume dairy, besides what Dr. Klaper mentions in his awesome video:

1. Dairy milk is high in phosphorous and low in magnesium, which your body needs to utilize calcium, so it's unable to absorb the calcium you think you're getting from milk!
2. Too much calcium in the body can lead to kidney stones, bone spurs, gout and atherosclerotic plaque.
3. Dairy milk may cause localized inflammation in the intestines of infants and that can lead to iron deficiency anemia.

Bottom line, move toward health by choosing dairy alternatives like the following:

- Organic, non-GMO almond, hemp or coconut milk (not soy).
- Make your own cashew cheese recipe (easy recipes online).
- Goat or sheep yogurt.
- Vegan ice cream (super yummy!).

Choose food that support the cells of your body. Dairy is NOT one of them!

Here are the approximate daily protein needs for kids and adults (developed by *New York Times* bestselling author Ocean Robbins, and Food Revolution Summit speaker Kris Carr):[19]

- Kids ages 4 to 13 = 0.43 grams.
- Adolescents ages 14 to 18 = 0.39 grams.
- Adults ages 19 to 64 (moderately active) = 0.36 grams.
- Seniors ages 65+ and special needs = 0.44 to 0.522 grams.

Are you ready for this next tidbit…Consume most of your protein in the evening. You don't need to consume it in the morning at all because your body needs energy at that time and should get it from unrefined carbohydrates and good fat. Eat protein more toward the end of the day to best support your body in repairing your tissue.

When you sleep, your body repairs itself and uses protein to do that. If you're still hungry after dinner, have a protein shake. There are many good ones on the market. Find one with under two grams of sugar, organic, non-GMO, with no artificial sweeteners or preservatives — and you'll be good to go! I recommend the vanilla flavored protein superfood by Amazing Grass. You can get it on Amazon. Buy two at a time and it will last you about twenty-two days. Protein shakes are

[19] Ocean Robbins (2019). Plant-Based Protein: What You Need to Know. [Article]. Retrieved from https://foodrevolution.org/blog/plant-based-protein/

an easy way to make sure you're getting adequate protein and they are great as an evening snack.

The third and final amazing food is unrefined carbohydrates.

Unrefined (Complex) Carbohydrates Versus Refined Carbs

You need carbohydrates to fuel your energy systems, and they are found in many types of foods. You've more than likely heard of complex and simple carbohydrates. I'd like you to think more about unrefined versus refined carbohydrates.

Unrefined carbs are a complete source of carbohydrates, which is found in real food, not processed food, and include natural sugars and fiber. Refined carbs are your simple carbs like white bread, enriched flour and refined sugar, which have had most nutrients removed and artificial ingredients added.

These foods are highly processed with little to no nutritional value. They are basically wasted calories!

When you eat unrefined carbs, you're telling your body to support your energy pathways, feed your good gut bacteria, optimize your metabolism, support your brain function and more!

Good sources of unrefined carbs include:

- Sweet potatoes
- Quinoa (substitute for rice or have as porridge in the morning)
- Cauliflower (substitute for rice)
- Veggies: leafy greens, broccoli, carrots
- Beans and legumes (also sources of protein)
- Nuts and seeds
- Fiber-rich fruit: apples, bananas, berries

Eating unrefined carbs in the morning for breakfast and lunch will support your energy systems and brain to give you what you need for your day! If you eat refined carbs in the morning, you'll be reaching for more sugar in the afternoon. It will spike your insulin making it nearly impossible for your body to burn fat. Plus, it will keep you stuck on the food addiction cycle.

How many unrefined carbs should you eat, and when? According to the Institute of Medicine, adult women should consume forty-five to sixty-five percent of their daily calories from carbohydrates:[20]

- 1,600-calorie diets need 180 to 260 grams.
- 2,000-calorie diets need 225 to 325 grams.

---

[20] Erin Coleman, R.D., L.D. (2018). The Recommended Intake of Grams of Carbohydrates per Day for Women. [Article]. Retrieved from https://healthyeating.sfgate.com/recommended-intake-grams-carbo-hydrates-per-day-women-5883.html

- 2,400-calorie diets need 270 to 390 grams.

Your body needs carbs for energy and many bodily functions. Start consuming the right kinds of carbs in the right amount and see how amazing you feel! When you eat food made out of refined sugars, you are telling your body to move toward disease.

You'll know if what you're eating is moving you toward health or disease by the following:

- How you feel
- Your energy levels
- Your focus and memory
- Your ability to release weight
- How your gut feels
- How your skin, hair and nails look

Here is a list of refined carbs to eliminate or reduce in your meal plan:

- Sodas
- Store-bought baked goods like muffins, cakes, pastries
- White bread
- Cereals

If you're going to eat refined carbs, be aware of how much you are eating. That is crucial to not only your waistline but your health. Your biggest concern should be your sugar intake.

The American Heart Association (AHA) recommends no more than 6 teaspoons (25 grams) of added sugar per day for women and 9 teaspoons (38 grams) for men. The AHA limits for children vary depending on their age and caloric needs, but ranges between 3–6 teaspoons (12–25 grams) per day.[21]

Remember, sugar is designed to trigger an addiction in your brain. If you are challenged with sugar cravings, your first step is to detox your body. That will release sugar cravings and help you drop inches easily. Then, start feeding your body unrefined carbohydrates, good fat and clean protein and you'll move toward health and release weight!

Food Timing and Combination

Do you remember a time when you were feeling great after dinner and then had dessert and knew that was too much? Proper food combining is **crucial**.

I've already quoted Raymond Francis in his book, *"Never Be Sick Again"* and this information is also based on his amazing book! He explains how certain foods digest differently in your body. If you eat them together, you'll end up with digestive issues. For example, your digestive system wasn't designed to

---

[21] Sugar Science, How Much Is Too Much? The growing concern over too much added sugar in our diets [Article] Retrieved from http://sug- arscience.ucsf.edu/the-growing-concern-of-overconsumption. html#. XPHcEi2ZPyI

break down protein and starches at the same time. Proteins digest in an acid environment and starches digest best in an alkaline environment. Eating them together will **hinder** your stomach's ability to break either of them down efficiently, which then does not allow your body to absorb the nutrients. This is the reason you feel bloated eating those foods together![22]

Vegetables can digest in either an acid or alkaline environment, so you can eat them with either proteins or starches. Yeah! Fruits digest quickly and should be eaten alone so they don't ferment in your gut, causing bloating and other digestive issues.

Another person I follow religiously is Dr. Joseph Mercola. I caught an interview he did with doctor, Dr. Wayne Pickering, which seconds what Raymond Francis is talking about. The following practice was taken from their interview on food combining. This way of eating will help you to easily release weight and feel great![23]

---

[22] Raymond Francis, M.Sc., Never Be Sick Again, Health Communications Inc. 2002, pp. 123-125

[23] Dr. Mercola. (2013). Dr. Mercola and Dr. Pickering Discuss Food Combining [YouTube Interview]. Retrieved from https://www.youtube.com/watch?v=fS8PY0RQcNw&t=75s

Practice: Food Combining and Timing

Here are the best food combinations that support your gut:

1. Eat protein with veggies and good fat.
2. Eat starches with veggies and good fat.
3. Eat fruit alone. (Eat acid fruits like grapefruit and oranges before sweet fruits like bananas and figs.)
4. Eat melons alone.
5. Eat dessert first (yeah!).

Did you see #4? If you love dessert, eat it first so your body can break down the sugar and it doesn't ferment in your gut. If you can, go for a twenty-minute walk and then have dinner; that would be perfect! Not only will your body feel a ton better, you won't feel guilty since you'll be burning off some of the sugar by walking… awesome!

Start eating how your digestive tract was designed and watch your health improve as you release inches and feel good about yourself! Oh yeah!

But wait, there's more…

The best food timing to support your energy, brain, hormones and weight loss:

- Breakfast: Fruit alone or with a protein/green shake, since it's already broken down.
- Lunch: Unrefined Carbs for lunch with veggies and good fat.
- Dinner: Protein and veggies for dinner with good fat.

Your energy system needs to fire-up first thing in the morning, so consuming sugar from fruit or unrefined carbs will give that system what it needs to get going. You still need energy in the early afternoon, and again, unrefined carbs are your best bet for that. In the evening, your body is slowing down and will repair itself when you sleep. That system needs protein to repair and rebuild tissue.

Throughout your day, you want to be supporting your fifty to seventy-trillion cells, so that is where good fat comes in! I take an Omega 3 supplement with most of my meals throughout my day to make sure my cells are getting what they need.

Yes, this way of eating is very different from the traditional way, and the traditional way is keeping you overweight and unhealthy!

Give this a try for a good thirty days and see how you feel. Be sure to have your smaller pair of jeans around because you'll be releasing inches like crazy!

I'd love to know how it goes for you or if you have questions. Post it on my Facebook page: Facebook. com/WomenBeingFit

Now that you know the best way to combine your food, here is the worst: sugary foods with protein, like a sweet dessert after a chicken or steak dinner, or a pastry with eggs, for breakfast. Those are seriously bad combinations for your gut!

When sugar and protein are combined, they form AGEs (advanced glycation end products). AGEs have been shown to promote a ton of health issues including heart disease, high blood pressure, arthritis, inflammation and more! Inflammation in your body makes it nearly impossible for you to release weight. The less inflammation you have, the better you will feel and the more you'll move toward health and release inches.[24]

You can get even more information on food combining and purchase an amazing food combining chart on Dr. Pickering's website...

Wayne-Pickering.com/HealthProducts/
FoodCombiningGuide.html

Lastly, your gut needs a break to empty from time to time. When your system is empty, it gives your cells the opportu-

---

[24] Raymond Francis, M.Sc., Never Be Sick Again, Health Communications Inc. 2002, p. 92

nity to clean house and detox. Think of it like a party where everyone (your cells) is mingling and enjoying food. When everyone leaves, you clean the house. Your body is no different. Your cells detox themselves when you don't have food in your system.

Here are five tips to support your gut on a regular basis:

Practice: Support Your Gut Health

1. Take a probiotic twenty minutes before breakfast or before you go to bed to give your gut good bacteria so it can easily break down the food you eat and your body can absorb the most nutrients. (Be sure you take it three-hours before or after any medications.)

2. Go twelve hours between your last meal and first meal of the day. This means have breakfast at 8 a.m. and don't eat anything after 8 p.m.

3. Wait for four hours between meals without snacks. (This one is challenging for me, so if I'm going to snack, I have either carbs with good fat or protein with good fat or just some good fat.)

4. Go for a ten-minute walk after meals to help your gut move things along.

5. Support your stomach enzymes by taking a digestive enzyme with most meals. (I use *Digestive Gold*. You can buy it on Amazon.)

Support your digestion in the best way you can, and you'll move toward health and easily release inches!

If you'd like help detoxing your body and want to learn even more about food, check out my *Boost Your Weight Loss* six-week program at WomenBeingFit.com/Detox

Don't be a slave to food manufacturers and their addictive foods. It's time to take back your power and feel and look your best! Now get ready for insights on cancer and what you can do to keep yourself safe.

Cancer Insights

I couldn't write a health book and not put insights I've learned about cancer. In 2006, I watched a dear aunt, who was more like a sister, transition out of her body from breast cancer. I stayed with her in the hospital for the last two weeks of her life. It was the hardest and most gratifying thing I've ever done.

I've wondered for a long time why our technology has changed so much over the past hundred years, but we are still using the same methods of dealing with cancer — chemo and radiation, that we've used over a hundred years ago.

I did a lot of digging and wanted to let you know things about cancer that are not commonly talked about in the mainstream. It is my hope they will be soon. Please use this information as education only. This isn't meant to cure anything. I encourage you to do your own research and give these supplements a try.

According to the Centers for Disease Control and Prevention, "Cancer is the second leading cause of death in the United States, exceeded only by heart disease. One out of every four deaths in the United States is due to cancer."[25] That is too many in my book, especially when the disease is preventable!

What Is Cancer?

Cancer is a mutated cell that multiplies, and your natural killer responses have been evaded or turned off. When cancer shows up, it is telling you one of three things: your environment or food and water are toxic, you are deficient in vitamins and minerals that your cells need to function optimally, or your emotions are mostly in the negative versus positive frequency.

---

[25] United States Cancer Statistics, (2015) Leading Cancer Cases and Deaths, Male and Female, 2015 [Statistics] Retrieved from https://gis.cdc.gov/Cancer/USCS/DataViz.html

It can also be telling you that all three things are happening at the same time: You are toxic, deficient in vitamins and minerals and have mostly negative, unloving feelings toward yourself and others.

Starting from birth, you've had mutated cells in your body. The great thing is that there is a part of your cellular system called apoptosis, which basically kills itself if something isn't functioning properly. Cancer evades or again turns off this system, and that's the problem!

When your cells are not filled with toxins, are getting the water and nutrients (vitamins and minerals) they need and you feel mostly content and happy in your life, then your immune system takes care of mutated cells and you don't get cancer.

However, if you are burning the candle at both ends, eating conventional processed foods, drinking sodas or tap water and other unfiltered water, feeling unloving thoughts on a daily basis you are moving your body toward disease and might be setting yourself up for cancer.

According to Dr. Leonard Coldwell, author of *The Only Answer To Cancer*, the root causes of cancer are:[26]

- Lack of energy
- Chronic stress

---

[26] The Answer to Cancer with Dr. Leonard Coldwell Beyond Belief with George Noory. (2013) Gaiam TV Original Episode

- Lack of self-love
- Compromising yourself
- Environmental issues
- Poor food and water quality

What I want to share next came from Dr. James Forsythe, who has been studying medicine since the 1950s; was the first oncologist in Reno, Nevada, and started the first three cancer wards there; was the head of the VA cancer program; the associate professor at the medical school in Nevada; and author of *Take Control of Your Cancer* and *Anti-Cancer Diet.*[27]

Dr. Forsythe's patients have a seventy-two percent survival rate of all cancer types. This is amazing, considering the survivor rate for Stage 4 cancer with conventional medicine is only around two percent after five years.

Here is what Dr. Forsythe does with each of his clients:

- Completes a cancer profile.
- Discovers what vitamins and minerals they are deficient in.
- Prescribes supplements to replenish needed vitamins and minerals.
- Detoxes to cleanse their system.
- Gets them on a clean diet.

---

[27] Full-Spectrum Cancer Therapy with James Forsythe, Healing Matrix with Regina Meredith. (2013) Gaiam TV Original Episode

- Uses oxygenation therapy (food-grade hydrogen peroxide).

Since 1911, we know that cancer cannot exist in an oxygen-rich and alkaline environment. This is why one of Dr. Forsythe's treatments is oxygenation therapy with food-grade hydrogen peroxide. You can get food-grade hydrogen peroxide online and do your own research to learn how to use it or better yet, find a doctor who can help you.

As I said earlier when I talked about sugar, cancer cells have more insulin receptors than regular cells, which means they take up sugar. Dr. Forsythe takes advantage of this and uses a Trojan Horse model, where he sends a small dose of chemotherapy with insulin into the body. The cancer cells think sugar is coming in and take the chemo into their cells. Since the chemo is going directly into the cancer cell, the side effects are greatly reduced. In a four-week period, he has seen a ninety percent reduction in tumors with this method. Awesome!

Dr. Forsythe also focuses on immune-boosting therapies when treating his patients. These include:

- Cutting out sugar and simple/refined carbohydrates.
- An alkaline diet (cancer creates acid and thrives in an acid environment).
- Eating detox foods such as garlic, beets, green organic veggies, wheat grass and broccoli.
- Drinking alkaline water to increase your PH.

- Juicing, which is a great way to get important nutrients in your body.
- Keeping processed foods to a minimum.
- Not Microwaving food in plastic containers, which can leach toxic compounds into your food.

Another helpful insight is not cooking with aluminum or Teflon cookware. That, too, can leach toxic compounds into your food, and Teflon has been shown to produce toxic fumes at high heat. Use stainless steel or other more high-end cookware. You're worth the investment. Also, don't wrap aluminum foil around hot or warm food. It can also leach toxic compounds into your food. You can keep yourself protected and heal from cancer in many ways that are within your control.

Cancer Tests

Be aware that some cancer tests can actually cause cancer! Your immune system is very sensitive to radiation. If you can, choose cancer tests that limit the amount of radiation you are subject to. For example, A CAT (CT) scan has 200 times the radiation of a simple chest X-ray. According to Consumer Reports, it is estimated that 15,000 people die each year because of cancers caused by the radiation in CT scans alone.[28]

I no longer get mammograms because I don't want to give my body radiation when I can ask for the Doppler method instead. The Doppler method uses high-frequency sound waves to view inside the body. Zero radiation.

I also do not go through the TSA screens at the airport. I get there early and ask to get a pat down. It doesn't take that much longer and eliminates one more way radiation enters my body. I use earbuds when I talk on my cell phone and I never, never, never sleep with my cell phone next to my head. That is a sure way to have small amounts of radiation affecting your brain as you sleep.

Only you can take responsibility for your health, and these easy tips can reduce your chances of cancer manifesting in your body.

Unfortunately, Big Pharma has a stake in keeping people sick, so there is a lot of misinformation out there. Don't take my word for it; do your own research and know the source of your research. If you find something that says food-grade hydrogen peroxide is bad, who is saying it? There is a lot of money in cancer treatments and as much as it saddens me to

---

[28] Consumer Reports, (2015), The surprising dangers of CT scans and X-rays. [Article] Retrieved from https://www.consumerreports.org/cro/magazine/2015/01/the-surprising-dangers-of-ct-sans-and-x-rays/index.htm

say, some big companies believe profit over people is what's important.

Here are some of the top cancer prevention supplements and natural ways I've found that you can protect yourself and support healing from cancer. Please do your own research and find out what's best for you.

Vitamin B-17: B-17 can be found in high amounts in apricot kernels and other seeds. According to G. Edward Griffin in his book, *World Without Cancer: The Story of Vitamin B17*, cancer cells produce an enzyme that "unlocks" the cyanide found in B17, which hinders and has been shown to stop the growth of cancer cells.[29]

Vitamin C: Vitamin C is an essential nutrient that supports your immune system. It has been shown to decrease cancer-related toxicities. Studies have shown that high-dose vitamin C decreased cancer growth in prostate, pancreatic, hepatocellular, colon, mesothelioma and neuroblastoma.

Vitamin D3: In a study conducted by Taiki Yamaji of the Center for Public Health Sciences of the National Cancer Center in Japan, she and her colleagues found people from Japan had a lower risk of cancer when they had higher levels

---

[29] A World Without Cancer (HQ) - The Story of Vitamin B17. Written by. G. Edward Griffin, 2012 [Documentary] Retrieved from [Documentary] Retrieved from https://www.youtube.com/ watch?v= sKhzbcpI_ro&t=107s

of Vitamin D. Vitamin D3 optimizes Vitamin D uptake in their bloodstream.[30]

Flor Essence Tea: This is a blend of herbs including burdock root, slippery elm, and more. It is a gentle, whole-body detox tea that is shown to boost your immune system, reduce inflammation, reduce chances of infection and provide pain relief. It also helps the body to eliminate toxins and may have anti-cancer properties. This tea can have strong side effects, so do your research to see if this is right for you.

Green Tea Extract: Decaffeinated green tea is a polyphenol antioxidant. It is a plant native to Asia, with antiviral and antioxidant properties that have been shown to protect your body against various cancers, including those of the prostate, stomach and esophagus.

IP-6: Inositol hexaphosphate (IP6) is a natural antioxidant found in many plants and vegetables high in fiber. You also have it in your cells. It supports your cells in communicating and functioning optimally. It has been shown to reduce the size of tumors and the spread of cancer. It also helps support your immune system, lowers cholesterol levels and maintains proper kidney function.

L-Glutathione: The most important antioxidant in the body, it is found in almost all of your cells and plays an

---

[30] Jasmin Collier, (2018) Vitamin D may protect against cancer [Article] Retrieved from https://www.medicalnewstoday.com/articles/321151.php

important role in detoxing carcinogens from your body. Studies have found that L-Glutathione prevents aging, heart disease, dementia and cancer. In fighting cancer, it supports your cells' apoptosis (cellular death) system.

Poly-MVA: This means multiple minerals, vitamins and amino acids. It protects and repairs your DNA and more importantly, your mitochondria, which is the energy of most of your cells and the source of cellular function. It also supports your cells' metabolism in keeping your cells functioning optimally.

Resveratrol: Resveratrol is an antioxidant found in red wine, grapes and some berries. Many in vitro and animal studies show that resveratrol inhibits cancer cell grown AND increases apoptosis, the system of cellular suicide.

Breathing: Oxygen is more critical to our bodies than any vitamin or mineral. If you don't breath correctly, your cells won't get a crucial element they need to run optimally and you'll actually change the chemistry in your body. Breathe correctly by bringing air into your diaphragm. In other words, breath into your belly the way you see babies breathing. Take slow, deep breaths through your nose for optimal oxygen consumption.

Sunlight: This is actually essential to your body's health as long as you're not getting burned. The DNA in your body is made of light! Your cells have light-activated receptors that can protect you from cancer. Studies show that proper sunlight helps regulate hormones, prevents infections, enhances the immune system, increases oxygen in your blood, nourishes and energizes your body.

According to Dr. Michael Holick, a professor of medicine, physiology and biophysics at the Boston University Medical Campus, to get optimal sunlight, allow ten to fifteen minutes or so of unprotected sun exposure to your arms, legs, abdomen and back. After that, follow up with good sun protection, like a 30 SPF or higher sunblock.[31]

Exercise: When you move your body, your cells detox and nutrients are delivered to them more efficiently. As scientist Raymond Francis says, "Exercise is like an essential nutrient; without it, your body malfunctions."[32]

Emotions: Your emotions may be contributing factor when it comes to cancer. In a paper published in the International Forum of New Science Oct 96: Effect of Conscious Intention on Human DNA, Dr. Glenn Rein, found that loving energy causes DNA to wind and heal, and negative energy causes DNA to unwind and die.[33] When you are having loving feel-

---

[31] Dr. Mercola, (2015) Sunlight — It Does Your Body Good [Article] Retrieved from https://articles.mercola.com/sites/articles/archive/2015/12/27/vitamin-d-sunlight.aspx

[32] Raymond Francis, M.Sc., Never Be Sick Again, Health Communications Inc. 2002, p.223

[33] Dr. Glen Rein, (2012) CHARACTERIZING THE EFFECT OF THE ENERGY EMITTED BY TRINFINITY8 ON HUMAN DNA [Article] Retrieved from https://www.trinfinity8.com/ research-dr-glen-rein/

ings you are helping your body repair and strengthen your immune system. Negative feelings are doing the opposite.

Water: Sixty percent of your body is water. You will die within three to four days if you don't drink water. It protects your tissue, spinal cord and joints; regulates body temperature; helps eliminate waste; helps in nutrient absorption and helps you lose weight! It is crucial to drink clean, filtered water. You should drink half your body weight in water a day. To get even more out of your water, add pink Himalayan salt, which will give you eighty-four trace minerals. You can learn more by researching, "Sole Water."[34] Dehydration kills your body. If you are thirsty, you're already dehydrated.

Lotions and Cleansers: Your skin is the largest organ of your body. It takes in particles of things you touch and put on it. Choose organic lotions, soaps and natural cleaners to limit your exposure to toxins.

As you can see, you can take many easy steps to supporting your body's cells and keeping yourself cancer free!

If you or someone you know is healing from cancer, the most important thing to do is optimize your nutrients to support your immune system. Maximum Green Vibrance is a great alkalizing protein shake. Take it as often as you can through-

---

[34] NDTV Food Desk, (2018) 5 Benefits of Starting Your Day With Himalayan Salt Water (Sole Water) [Article] Retrieved from https://food.ndtv.com/food-drinks/5-benefits-of-starting-your-day-with-himalayan-salt-water-sole-water-1728441

out your day and research the supplements mentioned here to see if they are right for you.

I don't like saying this, but a Western medicine doctor is not the best person for advice on healing from cancer. Their job is to treat the symptom, not the cause, and since they only have to take one nutrition class in their entire medical career, they don't understand the power of nutritional supplementation.

The Oncologist Story

I once took a friend to her oncologist and the doctor said that sugar does not feed cancer. My jaw about hit the floor and I wanted to grab my friend's hand and run us out the door! However, my friend was very scared. It was her cancer we were talking about and she trusted her doctor. Luckily, her treatment went well. She did maximize her nutrients to support her immune system, which I feel also supported her healing.

To learn more about how to heal and protect yourself or support someone you know who has cancer, here are three books I highly recommend:

- *Anti-Cancer Diet Book* by internationally acclaimed integrative medical oncologist James W. Forsythe, MD, HMD.
- *Take Control of Your Cancer* by James W. Forsythe, MD, HMD. Dr. Forsythe's cancer approach has

yielded a forty-six percent positive response rate in a five-hundred-patient study. Amazing!

- *The Only Answer to Cancer* by Dr. Leonard Coldwell, who has, to date, cured over 35,000 cancer patients (studies have concluded that he has a 92.3 percent cancer cure rate). He is one of the most endorsed naturopathic doctors in the world!

I also recommend you watch the documentary **The Truth About Cancer**. You will find it at TheTruthAboutCancer.tv

Cancer is a scary word and when you understand what it is and how to keep yourself protected, it doesn't have to be so scary. I'm looking forward to a world where cancer is a thing of the past! I know it can happen and you must be aware of what you're dealing with.

If you get cancer, don't just treat the symptom. Treat the cause! Like I said earlier, it can come from your environment, food and water, or emotions. Discover what it was and make the shift so you heal your cancer and limit your chances of getting it again.

These are the supplements I take on a daily basis to keep my cells running optimally and my body moving toward health:

- Perque Life Guard Multivitamin: Taken twice a day. One capsule in the morning and one in the afternoon.

- Perque EPA/DHA Guard (Omega 3): Taken with most meals.
- Physician's Choice Probiotic: Taken once a day before breakfast or before bed.
- Digestive Gold Enzymes: Taken with most meals.
- Vital Clear protein powder: Taken once or twice a day.
- Oolong tea: Drink in the morning.
- Filtered water: Drink forty to sixty-four ounces a day.

You can get all of these supplements on Amazon. However, don't go overboard. Add one supplement a month and see how you feel and always check with your doctor first. When looking at the cost, look at the per-serving price. For example, as of the time of this writing, a ninety-serving supply of Perque Life Guard Multivitamin is $1.05 a serving. It lasts for three months. It's worth it! Perque is an amazing company with some of the highest quality vitamins you can get! Look them up at https://www.perque.com.

I talked about Physician's Choice probiotics earlier. This supplement is super supportive for gut health and you don't need to take it all the time. If you regularly have two or more bowel movements a day, you can go off your probiotics. When you notice your bowel movements are no longer regular, go back on them.

Digestive Gold Enzymes are some of the best enzymes on the market. They support your stomach in breaking down food for better absorption and digestion.

Vital Clear protein powder contains a full range of vitamins and minerals, high-quality protein and fiber to help you stay satiated, promote liver function and help maintain healthy blood sugar levels.

I don't drink coffee anymore; I drink tea. It is not as acidic as coffee and has many health benefits. Plus, there are so many amazing flavors. You can even get many dessert teas. Yes, Oolong tea has caffeine, but it's not as much as coffee and doesn't give me that shaky, anxious feeling. Be sure you purchase organic, NON-GMO teas! It matters. Remember, toxins cause your cells to do weird things, so keep your food as clean as possible.

When you take supplements daily, you are supporting your cells, your body's energy systems, your brain function and more. My last tip on supplementing: Don't put your supplements in the cupboard! You will forget about them. Put them on the counter next to something you reach for every day. Get a small pill case and put the enzymes and EPA/DHA in it so you can carry them in your purse or wallet.

Put your probiotic next to your toothbrush and take it before you brush your teeth at night or after you use the restroom first thing in the morning. When your supplements are in view, you're more likely to take them and your money is well spent!

If you notice that your urine is bright yellow, that means you have **healthy** urine but you need to drink more water. I've heard that bright yellow urine is said to be "expensive" urine implying the brightness comes from the vitamins your body isn't absorbing. Yes, some of the vitamins will be lost in your urine but not all. Your body doesn't get the nutrients it needs from the food in the stores anymore. Those days are long gone. The soil isn't what it used to be and food manufacturing isn't what it used to be, either. Supplementation and eating more of a plant-based diet are your best chances if you want to make sure your body is getting what it needs nutritionally.

I recommended you use supplements for one month and see how you feel. If you don't feel any different, stop. My bet is you'll notice your energy, focus, memory, sleep and more improve. Start giving your body the nutrients it needs and it will love you for it!

Now that you have the inside of your body feeling better, let me tell you about the outside of your body. Oh yeah!

CHAPTER SEVEN

Get Fit for Your Body type

When you understand how to train and eat for your body type, it will be a lot easier to get quick and lasting results.

In the 1940s, American psychologist William Sheldon popularized three general body type categories: ectomorph, mesomorph, and endomorph. An ectomorph body has a small frame, mostly thin. This body type is challenged to build muscle. A mesomorph body has a medium frame, a thick strong body, and it builds muscle easily. It can be challenged with weight but can release it fairly quickly. An endomorph body has a large frame, soft body and is challenged with excess body fat because of its slower metabolism.

You may have traits of more than one body type, but your body's metabolism and shape are dominant to one. You'll want to train for that body type.

Here are keys to knowing your dominant body type:

- If you're mostly round and releasing weight is challenging, train and eat for an endomorph body type.
- If you're challenged to gain muscle and are mostly thin, train for an ectomorph body type.
- If you can gain and lose weight fairly quickly and if you build muscle easily, train for a mesomorph body type.

The majority of my clients have an endomorph body type. Here is the link to a **free quiz** I created so you can find out what body type you have https://womenbeingfit.com/fitnessquiz/

Body Types and What You Need to Know

Mesomorph

Some would say that a person with a mesomorph body type drew the long straw. However, I feel that you choose the body you are in for emotional expansion toward love and forgiveness of yourself and others, so I believe all the body types have gifts and lessons to teach us. I know you are in the most perfect body for your emotional growth in this lifetime. Oh yeah!

Examples of women with a mesomorph body type include:

- Sarah Jessica Parker
- Tina Turner
- Jennifer Garner
- Madonna
- Gloria Estefan
- Halle Berry

Mesomorph physical body traits include:

- Naturally lean, muscular and strong
- Athletic physique
- Medium size joints/bones
- Broad/square shoulders
- Hourglass figure
- Tones up easily
- Releases weight fairly quickly

Your body can look lean or muscular. It's really your choice and depends on how you train and eat. You build muscle easily, so if your goal is to stay lean and toned, cardio should be your focus. When thinking of cardio, think easy, flat long runs. If you choose hills or intensity training, you could build up your thighs and calves. If you want that, go for it! If not, stick with slow-pace, long cardio workouts, and you'll lean up.

A friend of mine who has a mesomorph type body took dance classes and spent hours training. She trained at an easy/

medium pace and her body was amazingly lean and toned even though she didn't lift any weights!

Here is an example of a workout schedule for a mesomorph:

- Monday: 40–60-minute easy jog or Zumba class
- Tuesday: Endurance toning with light weights
- Wednesday: 40–60-minute easy jog or Zumba class
- Thursday: Yoga (optional)
- Friday: Endurance toning with light weights
- Weekends: Off or an easy jog or Zumba class

The strength training practices in my *Be Fit* online workout program will help you tone up but not bulk up, especially if you only use three-to five-pound weights. As long as you don't use heavy weights, nearly ANY activity will allow you to release weight and tone up!

Do a minimum of two cardio sessions a week, and all in moderation. You can also do cardio and strength training in the same workout or split them up and do one day of strength and the next day of cardio. If you want to build more muscle, focus on heavier weights and lower reps. You get to decide!

The next body type has more of a challenge building muscle. However, they always look fairly thin so have the illusion of being fit, even if they haven't worked out in years!

Ectomorph

Examples of women with an ectomorph body type include:

- Kate Moss
- Audrey Hepburn
- Cameron Diaz
- Models
- Michelle Melendez (me)

Ectomorph body traits include:

- Thin
- Small joints/bones
- Long arms and legs
- No hips (rectangle shape)
- Small shoulders
- Small chest and buttocks
- Low body fat (without exercising or following low-calorie diets)
- Difficulty gaining weight and muscle
- Lots of energy

Since gaining muscle is a challenge, if that is your goal, you should up your protein intake, especially on the days you strength train. You'll want to eat at least .7 grams of protein per pound of body weight. So if you want to be 120 pounds, you should eat eighty-four grams of protein a day.

If you want to build muscle, you MUST strength train! You should do a minimum of two days of strength training a week, and preferably three! You can do either endurance toning, meaning medium weight and longer repetitions, or if you REALLY want to see results, do heavier weights where you can only lift the weight for eight to twelve reps before your muscle feels burned out. I do both of these types of workouts two to three times a week, sometimes on the same day, and I don't looked buffed at all!

Ectomorphs have smaller joints, so the best way to train is with a bit heavier weights and fewer reps to keep your joints happy. Joints tend not to like lots of repetition.

Here is an example of what I do...

I teach endurance toning workout classes twice a week. On some days, I'll lift fifteen-pound free weights eight to twelve times for three to six sets right after class. Yep, that's fifteen pounds for each arm. I do that at least twice a week! That keeps my arms firm but it would take even more days of training to really bulk them up.

That's an ectomorph body type. It's challenged to build muscle. Just is what it is. Your goal should be to bring your muscles to fatigue by the end of your set, which means you are feeling the muscle burn. You also feel a bit sore the next day. If you don't, you're wasting your time! The strength training and cardio exercises on my *Be Fit* online workout program would be perfect for you!

Cardio workouts alone are not a great way for you to get the results you want. Don't get me wrong; in terms of overall health, being fit and feeling great, cardio is important! Still, a lot of ectomorphs use cardio as their go-to exercise and it really should be strength training.

When you do cardio, do the infamous HIIT (high-intensity interval training) to increase your fitness level and endurance and feel the high that only comes from a good workout! Long cardio days are over unless you're training for a marathon, or you enjoy them.

Long cardio workouts burn both fat AND muscle, and if your goal is to tone up, that is not the workout for you! Your workouts should be strength training eighty percent of the time. You don't have to do a sixty-minute workout. Twenty to thirty minutes will be perfect, plus, you only need to do cardio once or twice a week. The other workouts should be strength training.

Here is an example of a workout schedule for an ectomorph:

- Monday: Endurance toning with medium weights
- Tuesday: 30–40-minute HIIT cardio practice
- Wednesday: Endurance toning with medium weights
- Thursday: Yoga or another 30–40-minute HIIT cardio practice
- Friday: Endurance toning with medium weights
- Weekends: Off or throw in a Yoga class

If you have an ectomorph body, give that workout schedule a shot and watch as your body tones up and feels great!

Have you've been struggling with your weight most of your life? You more than likely have an endomorph body type.

Endomorph

Examples of women with an endomorph body type include:

- Jennifer Lopez
- Beyoncé
- Marilyn Monroe
- Oprah Winfrey
- Queen Latifah
- Kate Winslet
- Roseanne Barr

Even though your body can be challenged with excess weight, you can still look amazing! Marilyn Monroe had an endomorph type body... hello!

Traits of an endomorph body type:

- Smooth, round body (can be solid or doughy)
- Medium/large joints/bones
- Narrow or small shoulders
- Short limbs
- Struggles with excess body fat and weight loss

- Carries excess weight in lower regions of body, mainly lower abdomen, butt, hips and thighs
- Can have pear-shaped or hourglass body
- Can gain muscle easily, but you can't tell
- Slower metabolism
- May get tired easily
- Falls asleep easily but may have trouble staying asleep

The biggest challenge with this body type is the slower metabolism. That means you'll burn less calories when at rest than the other two body types. In other words you hold on to fat very easily. Your focus MUST be on increasing your metabolism naturally, and the two keys for that are building more lean muscle and eating a diet low in refined carbs and sugar. Odds are you already know this.

Your nutrition is key more than for any of the other body types. It is eighty percent of your success. Actually, ninety percent of your success will come from releasing your emotional addiction to struggling with your weight, and nutrition is the second key to your success.

You should do a minimum of two days of endurance strength training a week, and preferably three. Do not lift heavy weights or you could build larger muscles and look bigger versus leaner.

Endurance toning type exercises, meaning medium to light weights and longer repetitions, should be your go-to workouts. You'll want to bring your muscles to failure by the end of your set, which means you are feeling your muscle burn and you feel a bit sore the next day. You don't need to overdo it, but you do need to feel that you did some work.

If you feel so sore you can barely move, you overdid it. You should feel tight muscles and be able to go throughout your day without it being too much of a distraction.

Many women with this body type enjoy walking. Walking is wonderful to begin with and if you want results, you must strength train as often as possible and honor your body with good nutrition.

Here is an example of a workout schedule for an endomorph:

- Monday: 30–40-minute endurance toning with light/medium weights
- Tuesday: 20–40-minute HIIT cardio practice
- Wednesday: 30–40-minute endurance toning with light/medium weights
- Thursday: 20–40-minute yoga, or rest
- Friday: 30–40-minute endurance toning with light/medium weights
- Saturday: 20–40-minute HIIT cardio practice
- Sunday: 20–40-minute Yoga, or rest

Since your metabolism is slower than the other body types you'll want to do some kind of exercise almost daily. Plus, again you absolutely MUST do endurance strength training workouts! That will help increase your metabolism right away.

Decide what days you'll do your strength training and cardio practices and put a reminder on your cellphone. For a fun endurance toning workout that includes affirmations of self-acceptance, go to www.WomenBeingFit.com/FunWorkout. You'll love it!

The Intensity of Your Workout

Before you start any exercise program, check with your doctor to make sure you are cleared to workout. The intensity of your workout is crucial! As I said earlier, most women will go for a walk. Walking is a great place to start, and after you've been walking for four to six weeks, it's time to pick up the pace!

In order to get the results you want with your workouts, you must understand your intensity scale.

Intensity Scale:

1 2 3 4 5 6 7 8 **9 10**
Very Easy **Challenging Very Hard**

Here is what it will look like: Start your workout in the lighter zone and spend three to five minutes warming up. After that, you want to start feeling your heart rate beating a bit more.

You're beginning to sweat and your breath is getting quicker. You can talk but it feels challenging to do so. This is a level seven intensity in the medium zone. Now, stay here for about two to three minutes.

To burn the most calories for your fitness level, increase your intensity quickly by doing an interval where you get your heart rate to a level eight or nine on the intensity scale for thirty-seconds up to a minute, and that's it! That will put you in the darker zone.

In the darker zone, you'll be sweating, feel challenged, it will be hard for you to talk and you really don't want to be there. Don't worry, you'll only be there for thirty to sixty-seconds, max!

After your interval, take the intensity back to either the lighter or medium zone and repeat that cycle at least two to three times per workout. This is how you can make a twenty-minute workout burn more calories than a sixty-minute workout!

My *Burn Your Fat, Free Your Heart* cardio practices could be tremendously beneficial for you! These workouts are designed to not only burn your fat, they free your heart of worry, stress, negative self-talk or ANY negative emotion! They leave you feeling good in your body and feeling great about yourself! For a free *Burn Your Fat, Free Your Heart* cardio workout, visit www.WomenBeingFit.com/BurnFatCardio. You can download that workout to your iPod or iPhone and listen as you do any cardio activity.

If you'd like to share with me how your first workout goes for you, please post a comment on Facebook at Facebook.com/WomenBeingFit. I'd love to hear from you.

My Getting in Shape Story

When I first started working out, I thought I was going to throw up and die. No joke! Before I became a fitness instructor, I sold gym memberships. I knew I needed to get in shape if I was going to be good at sales, so I thought I would go for a run up the nearby hill and come back down. By the time I got back, I was as red as a tomato and wanted to puke my guts out.

I even asked my friend who was the aerobics director, "Am I the only one who feels like they are going to die after they run up a hill for the first time, or is that everyone?" Her reply, "Nope, that's everyone."

I'm living proof that regular exercise doesn't stay so challenging. It gets easier. I've been teaching fitness for nearly twenty years now, and a few years back I had a new client ask me if it will always hurt. The answer is yes but the pain changes.

Remember when I said that you create new cells every two months? Well, those new cells will actually function more optimally because of your workouts, so the discomfort you feel will not be the same as when you started.

Your workouts get easier roughly every four to six weeks. However, there will always be a level of discomfort, or you won't see any changes in your body. The body needs to get uncomfortable for change to happen and to maintain the benefits you have from your current workouts.

What's amazing about the body is that it will want to adapt to the new discomfort, and as long as you're eating the right foods, your body will burn your fat to feed your muscle. Isn't that wonderful?! Your body is seriously amazing!

When starting your exercise regimen, start slowly. If you go too hard too soon, you could get discouraged and give up! Don't let that happen to you. Slower is better!

Beginner Workout

Here is a beginner workout that will get you going slowly. It works nearly all of your upper and lower body muscles in only two strength training exercises.

Week One and Two:

- Do two ten to twenty-minute **walks**.
- Once or twice during the week, do thirty-seconds up to one-minute **Table Push-ups and Chair Squats**

Table Push-Ups (Thirty-Seconds):

- Put your hands on the table a little wider than your shoulders.
- Stand about three feet away from the table.
- Keep your shoulders down and bring your chest as close to the table as you can without touching it. (You should be looking up toward the middle of the table and not at the floor.)
- Inhale on the way down and exhale as you push back up.
- Repeat at a consistent **and** comfortable pace doing as many as you can in thirty-seconds.
- Be sure to count so you know the number you need to meet or beat the next time you do it.
- Stretch your chest for at least fifteen to thirty-seconds. To learn how, go to YouTube and do a search for "easy chest stretches."

Chair Squats:

- Put a chair behind you as if you're going to sit on it.
- Act like you're going to sit but don't. Go down about halfway or wher-

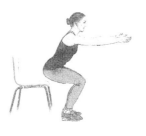

ever you can easily stand back up **without** touching the chair.

- Reach your arms away from you and press your hips back, making sure your knees are **behind** your toes and **not** in front.
- Repeat at a consistent **and** comfortable pace doing as many as you can in thirty to sixty-seconds.
- Be sure to count so you know the number you need to meet or beat the next time you do it.
- Inhale on the way down and exhale on the way up.
- Stretch your quads and hamstrings for 15-30 seconds each. To learn how, go to YouTube and do a search for "easy stretch quads and hamstrings."

Week Three: Do Table Push Ups and Chair Squats one time each. Rest for thirty to sixty-seconds and repeat so you're doing two-sets. Also, halfway through your walk, do an interval by picking up the pace and going as fast as you can for fifteen to thirty-seconds. Then, return back to your walk.

Week Four and Five: Add another interval to your walk when you're about four-minutes toward completion. Increase the time of your chair squats and table push-ups by ten to fifteen-seconds during both sets.

Week Six: Try one of my Level One workouts from my *Be Fit* online workout program or any beginner ten to twenty-minute full body workout online! Now you're ready!

Always keep track of your workouts either manually with a calendar or with a phone app. There are so many fun and easy ways to track your workouts. I even have a fun app on my *Be Fit* program. Tracking helps you to stay motivated and is a fun way to watch yourself progress.

Prepare for Your Workout the Night Before

To be the MOST successful, prepare the night before your workout. If you're going to the gym, prepare your gym bag and place it by the door. If you're doing your exercise at home, know the time you'll workout and get the area ready the night before or as soon as you can. Then, get excited that you get to do the workout! Think about your heart-based goal and how great it's going to feel achieving it! Before you go to bed, really sit with the feelings of excitement and the joy you'll have living your heart-based goal. Let those feelings pull you out of bed the next morning to do your workout! Oh yeah!

You Don't Have to Workout… You Get To!

Here is another tip that will help you stay inspired to workout. When thinking of doing a workout, don't think that you have to workout, think that you get to workout.

Who likes doing things they have to do? If you're like me, I'd rather do things that I get to do. Things you have to do include:

- Taking out the garbage
- Doing the dishes
- Doing the laundry
- Washing the dog

If you get to do something, that makes it way more exciting! Things that you get to do include:

- Going to Disneyland
- Going to the movies
- Going out to dinner
- Going to a party

You get the picture. When you get to do something, it is much more fun than if you have to do something.

Practice: You Get to Workout!

Think about your next workout and get excited that you get to do it!

Lay out your clothes and leave them in the bathroom where you're going to change. Have your water bottle, towel and purse all next to the front door if you're going to the gym.

If you're doing one of my *Be Fit* online workouts or working out with me live, have your exercise mat, free weights and fit ball ready to go near your computer or TV, wherever you'll be doing your workout.

The night before, get excited that you're going to do your workout the next day... like REALLY excited! Think about your heart-based goal and get excited that you get to experience that very soon in your life!

Let your heart-based goal be the catalyst that pulls you to get up and do your workout!

You don't have to do your workout... you get to! Oh yeah! It's all a game and you get to make up the rules. Start having more fun with your life. You deserve it!

If you play this game, it will change the way you think about exercise. What if, in a few short months, you were working out regularly and enjoying it? You even looked forward to it! That's possible for you!

You are only addicted to thinking about exercise the current way you do because you've memorized thinking about it like that. Play a game that will help you shift and watch as you get in shape and start feeling great about your body!

Are you curious why you got stuck with a life journey of struggling with your weight? If you've ever said, "Why me?!" then the next chapter was written for you!

CHAPTER EIGHT

The Purpose of Your Lifetime Struggle with Weight

Why are you here in the first place? What is the purpose of it all? Why has your struggle with weight been so hard for so long?

When you emotionally expand and move toward love and forgiveness of yourself and others, and REALLY live it, feeling it in every cell of your body, you evolve into a new higher vibrational version of yourself, and that not only changes your life but also helps change the world for the better!

Emotionally expanding toward love and forgiveness helps humanity evolve toward peace, which is the next step for humankind.

Your journey has been so hard for so long because the next phase of human evolution is peace and love, and most of us are way off track! The vibration that humanity holds today is not lined up with our next step in evolution, and we feel it in every cell of our bodies!

Instead of peace, there is still a billion or even trillion dollar budget for wars. The media feeds you lies about what is beautiful, and you buy it. Instead of loving yourself and others, you are brainwashed to love things. Are you on the roller-coaster ride of consumerism?

One of my favorite quotes is, *"The best things in life aren't things."* — *Author unknown.* If that was the world's motto, you would be living in a body you love right now! When you compare yourself with others, when you don't feel grateful for what you have, when you don't feel good enough by just being you, your journey with weight never ends.

It's time to understand that YOU are part of the evolution of the Universe. You haven't always been here on Earth and you're not staying for more than eighty to a hundred years or less.

Your higher-self or soul, whatever you want to call it, decided to come to earth and experience life in your human body and emotionally expand through your experiences and the emotional addictions your ego created from your past. It did that to create the next step in human and universal evolution. That is the purpose of your lifelong struggle with weight.

Scientists now believe that the Universe is conscious and is constantly evolving and expanding. That means you and everything around you are constantly evolving and expanding. The evolution of our species hasn't stopped! The next stage of evolution is an awakening to who we are and emotionally moving toward love and forgiveness of ourselves and others.

Nicolas David Ngan has this to say about the consciousness of the Universe… "One of the ways the Creative Force of the Universe seeks to expand its consciousness is to separate parts of itself. These parts (us) forget that they are part of the whole. The purpose of dropping into the forgetfulness of separation consciousness is that we experience life through a particular set of ego personality filters. We initially believe that this (our life) is all that is. We re-experience ourselves as ALL that is through specific life lessons to expand the consciousness of ALL that is."[35]

There is an intelligence inside you that lives in every cell of your body. It keeps your heart beating, your immune system running, your muscles contracting and expanding, your food digesting and so on. It's doing it all without a to-do list on your part!

This intelligence organizes tens of thousands of chemical reactions in every cell of your body per second every day. You

---

[35] Nicolas David. Ngan, Your Soul Contract Decoded. New York: Osprey Publishing, 2013. p. XX

don't plug yourself into a wall or use electricity to run your body. This intelligence is the electricity!

Why Is This Important?

Do you think it's an accident that you're in the body you're in, that you have the parents you have, that you were born in the town you were born in, that you've experienced the trauma and the joys you've experienced, or even that you have the career you have? No, friend, there is an intelligence that put you here to be YOU! Exactly as you are! - with all your funny, odd and beautiful parts.

That same intelligence put the planets in orbit; runs the tides in the ocean; informs butterflies, birds and whales where to migrate, and so on. It also put you on a journey toward self-love which begins with transforming your emotional addiction from the feeling of struggling with your weight to ending dieting hell and living in a body you love!

Look at your entire life as though you're watching a movie and see how it flows. Can you see the river of your life with its rapids and calm waters? Can you see that even the most challenging thing you've been through was meant to move you toward love and forgiveness? Whether you chose to go there or not was up to you.

I look back at my own life, and I remember when I hired a trainer to teach a class and she stole the clients from me. It took me months to stop being angry and forgive her, and when I did, I was inspired to move my business where I really wanted it to be, which was online. I now live on the Big Island of Hawaii and have an online business that I love and had been a dream for more years than I can remember!

The things that happened in your life, including people and events, were all meant for one thing... to move you toward self-love and forgiveness. When you allow yourself to experience that, you'll finally get what you want, which is peace, and the weight will release from your body. Judging and struggling against the way things are make your life journey very challenging and you miss messages and inspirations trying to come to you.

It's not a mistake you're receiving this information now at this time in your life. You are ready for the next phase of your emotional evolution. Like I said in an earlier chapter, you are the evolution of your family. Your father was the evolution of his parents. Your grandfather the evolution of his parents, and so on.

Look at it this way... parents normally want more for their children monetarily than they had in their lives. This is the same when it comes to emotional expansion. Your parents and grandparents may have dealt with the same issue of struggling with their weight, like you are. However, you have the opportunity to end the cycle and bring you and your family peace.

If you choose to emotionally expand to live in a body you love, it will be the next evolutionary sequence in your family line and you will not only heal yourself but those who came before you will experience the healing on a vibration level, too.

Healing Ancestry Line Story

I was visiting a friend who was a pyschic and we were talking about my anger issue. Even though I had good cause to have created my anger addiction, I didn't know that it was ancestral. I knew my father had anger issues, but I didn't know that my grandfather or great-grandfather also struggled with anger. It came up when I was doing a healing session. I could feel in my heart and intuition that the anger started with my great-grandfather having been in a war. He felt powerless and emotionally attached to anger. It was so intense that it went down the generation line to me.

Feeling powerless was my experience many times when I would feel angry. That pattern was very familiar to me. When I healed that part of me in the session, I felt it move through my family line and a feeling of relief came over me like a weight had been lifted.

I later asked a family member if my great-grandfather was ever in a war. She told me he was from Chihuahua and Durango and was around at the time of the Mexican crusaders, which overthrew the dictator of forty years, Porfirio Diaz, in 1910, so he very well could have been a part of that conflict.

If your parents and grandparents have struggled with weight, then they built the cocoon and you are meant to emerge as the butterfly. It's the natural evolution toward the next step if you choose to elevate your emotional frequency toward love and forgiveness. If not, you will stay at a lower emotional frequency like frustration, and feel stuck forever!

My hope for you is that you choose to emotionally expand toward love and forgiveness. That is the energy your consciousness came from and where it will return to when you transition out of your body.

The Universe started with the frequency of love. It's in everything around you, including every one of your seventy-plus trillion cells! This is why it feels so good to love. It's because it returns you to your natural state of being. It's also the reason negative feelings feel so bad. They move your energy away from your natural state of being, and that is very unpleasant.

Your job is to let go of who you think you are (ego) and surrender your story that you are someone who struggles with weight. I hope by now you realize that is not who you are. That is only a memorized emotional addiction that feels normal and familiar but it is far from who you are.

Practice: Get to Know the Intelligence Inside You

Put your hand on your heart and ask, "What is the intelligence that knows how to expand and contract my lungs and beat my heart?"

Go to the bathroom and look in the mirror. Look into your left eye, which is over your heart, and FEEL the intelligence inside you looking back at you with complete love and appreciation for your journey in life.

Go outside and feel the sun shining on your face. The same intelligence inside you put the sun in the sky in the exact location so the earth could sustain life and you could feel its warmth.

Finally, ask this intelligence for a sign that it is you. Then open your heart and trust something is showing up that will show you.

When I asked for a sign that infinite intelligence was with me, I saw a monarch butterfly fly right in front of me. That meant a lot to me because I used to live near a grove where thousands of monarchs would congregate and mate once a year. It was amazing!

Your life is so much more than your relationships, events and circumstances. Yet, that is where you need to start in order to feel the abundance that surrounds you. You have to start by fully **accepting** all of your life exactly the way it is and has been. Create a loving relationship with the younger parts of you and welcome each emotion you have without making it wrong. That will bring you the peace you so deserve and are ready for.

Yes, it's been challenging, but your journey toward a body you love means more than you know. It will help change the world and move us all toward peace, and the world is ready and needs that more than ever!

I've given you many practices to shift your emotional frequency and help you emotionally expand. Here is another one...

Practice: Ask for Help

Ask the infinite intelligence that put you here for help.

You are a unique version of the Universe and your journey toward experiencing peace in your body is unlike any other person's on the planet or in history! Because of the law of free will, infinite intelligence can only help if you ask.

When you get stuck, use my *Live in a Body You Love* prayer to ask the Universe for help. Here it is again...

Live in a Body You Love Prayer:

Guides, Angels, Source of All Things…I know I'm on an emotional healing and awakening journey with my body. Please help me find compassion for all I've been through. Inspire me to choose foods, thoughts and actions that nourish my body and soul. Help me live in peace in a body I love.
Thank you,
Amen.

If you're stuck and having a challenging day, say this prayer and then get into the present moment. That will increase your vibrational frequency and you can choose your next action and thought. Open your heart and trust the inspirations that show up.

Business Story

A while back, I didn't know what the next step was for *Women Being Fit*. Before I went to bed that night, I asked the intelligence inside me to tell me my next step. At 4:30 a.m., I woke up and knew I was supposed to do a teleseminar. I was so excited that I couldn't go back to sleep. The teleseminar was a huge success!

The reason inspiration hit me at 4:30 a.m. was because my conscious mind was not in the way of the message wanting to come through.

When you are in judgment of yourself or others, stressed or worried about life, messages from your higher-self and inspirations cannot reach you. One way to help you hear them during your day is to get in the present moment.

The present moment is a magical place that very few people utilize. When you pause in the middle of an emotion and get into the present moment, you create space between your reactions and emotions. You can then decide what you want to think instead of having your memorized patterns run your life!

Practice: The Magic of the Present Moment!

The next time you notice yourself feeling something negative about your body, do the following:

- Focus on your breath.
- Feel the different temperatures that surround your body.
- Hear the sounds in the room and beyond.
- Notice how you're sitting or standing.
- Feel the boundary of your clothes on your body.

Ask yourself who is breathing me? Who is beating my heart? Who is seeing through my eyes?

> Notice everything that makes up your present moment. This will give your body a break from your own self-talk and judgments, and start to return you back to a relaxed state.
>
> When you focus on the loving intelligence beating your heart and breathing you, you'll open up to the magic of who you are. You can then choose what you want to think and feel and get to know yourself as someone who lives in a body you love. That is the power of who you are!

I want to give you another tip from my Live in a Body You Love program that is super fun and allows the infinite intelligence inside you to work through your life and bring you miracles!

Get Curious

A simple inquiry I use all the time, especially when I am dealing with a challenging situation, is… *"I'm curious to see how this is going to work out. I know things always work out for me and I'm curious to see who I'm going to meet and what events are going to happen to have everything work out for me."*

This next story is really fun and shows how I use this inquiry.

Husky Puppy Story

I was on a reality TV show in Alaska. The show was about doing things that people have on their bucket list, like riding quads (an all terrain vehicle) to an ice glacier, river rafting, and taking an off-road Jeep tour. You get the picture.

One event that I was REALLY looking forward to was going to see the husky puppies at the Husky Homestead. The Husky Homestead raised dogs to race in the Iditarod Race, which is nearly a thousand-mile race over the most beautiful and challenging terrain in the world! The leader of our crew was supposed to set it up for us to visit, but by Wednesday, it still wasn't set up. Every time I asked him when we were going to see the puppies, either he hadn't yet contacted them or they hadn't gotten back to him. Our crew was set to leave on Saturday and it was Thursday night!

I paused and thought... okay, I know everything I want shows up in ways I know and in ways I don't know. I'm curious to see how we are going to see the husky puppies and I'm open to it happening in whatever way it wants. I then got really excited to see the puppies AND really curious how it was going to work out.

The next day, our last day in the area, we were set to go on a Jeep tour. When we got there, they weren't ready for us and told us to go for a ten- to fifteen-minute walk. I walked to the first house in the area, and these two beautiful huskies ran over to me, wagging their tails.

I looked at the owner, standing on his porch, and asked if I could pet his dogs. He smiled and said, "Yes." I then told him how my group was trying to go and see the puppies at the Husky Homestead but they hadn't gotten in touch with us yet.

He said… are you ready for this… "My daughter is in charge of setting up groups to go there. She went to the store and will be back in twenty minutes."

What?! I started screaming and jumping up and down. We went to see the puppies the next morning and it was awesome!

Don't let your mind fool you! It just takes practice! Being curious is an AMAZING tool to release stress and let the Universe bring you what you want! When you are curious, your subconscious mind cannot negate it. Isn't that awesome?!

When you say, "I'm curious how it will feel when I'm confident without my clothes and the lights on or off!" There's nothing to negate! It's simply an inquiry of curiosity.

Your unconscious mind wants to please you so it's going to find feelings and stories it can show you in your mind of what it might be like doing that. This is so fun! It's the backdoor to getting what you want and it's easy to do!

Your life is a game of experiences that touch your heart and challenge your soul. The end-game is to move toward love and forgiveness of yourself and others. Doing that allows your spirit to emotionally expand, which increases the vibration of the entire planet and helps us all evolve to our next level of humanity, which is again, peace.

You're not the stories you keep telling yourself about your limitations and how you're not good enough. Those are only lower vibrational frequencies that you're addicted to and that your body has memorized. They are not who you are and they don't have to be who you become.

You've had a challenging life, sweet friend. Being alive at this time in history takes courage, strength and trust. Your courage comes from the fact that you survived your childhood and have a pretty decent life right now, or you wouldn't be reading this. Your strength comes from your desire to create change and be happy. Your trust comes from the knowledge that there is something greater than your mind that is supporting you.

Infinite intelligence wanted to experience life in your body, as you, having gone through everything you've gone through. Why? Because there has never been anyone like you in all of history, nor will there ever be anyone like you again. You are a unique expression of infinite intelligence.

When you dislike your body and put yourself down, you don't allow yourself to grow and you will stay stuck in a body you don't love for the rest of your life!

Your hardest job will be to stop making yourself wrong and let go of wishing things could be different in your life. Start accepting all you've been through and trust it was supposed to happen that way, even if it SUCKED!

I'm sure you understand now that diet and exercise programs will never work for you if you don't allow yourself to release your emotional addiction to the feeling of struggling with your weight. Don't get me wrong. Diet and exercise programs do work. However, if you have been struggling with your weight year after year for most of your life, they are NOT the answer for you until you first release your emotional addiction to the feeling of struggling with your weight!

You have a choice to make… do you want to evolve into the next phase of yourself or do you want to stay in what is comfortable and familiar and let your ego continue its patterns of self-loathing because that's what it knows and with which it is comfortable?

If you want to stay struggling with your weight and body image, you can do that for the rest of your life, and many people do.

It's Your Free Will and Your Right to Choose.

However, if you choose to expand your spirit, grow-up emotionally and release your memorized addictions that keep you stuck with weight you don't want, you will create a new way of being in the world and feel an enormous freedom in your life.

You can't go back now that you know this information. It has forever changed you. It's time to listen to your body and start a dialogue with the infinite intelligence inside you that wants you to emotionally expand and evolve to the next level of your human experience.

When you start to communicate with this intelligence and ask it for help when you need it, you will feel new inspirations that move you toward a body you love. This intelligence has been waiting for you to wake up to who you are and communicate with it. It has so many insights to share with you to make your journey in this life meaningful, fulfilling, easy and joyful! You can do it. It only takes practice. There is a very special prayer that ancient Hawaiians have used for centuries that can help you. I want to end this book by teaching it to you.

CHAPTER NINE

Ancient Hawaiian Prayer: Ho'oponopono

The ancient Hawaiians have a prayer of forgiveness that allows them to come back into harmony with their community, family and friends. This prayer is called Ho'oponopono.

"Ho'o" means to make and "pono" means right. Stating it twice means to make double right. Here are the simple words of this prayer:

I'm sorry.
Please forgive me.
Thank you.
I love you.

Yes, they are simple words and they were part of a sacred foundation of harmony the Hawaiians valued for hundreds of years.

This prayer is not only intended to bring people back in harmony with themselves and each other for wrongdoings, but also to bring humanity peace, which, like I said earlier, is the next phase of our evolution. Ho'oponopono is always, and only, for yourself — never for anyone or anything else!

A dear friend of mine here on the Big Island of Hawaii does workshops to teach people the life-changing practice of Ho'oponopono. Here is what he has to say: "Over a decade of practicing Ho'oponopono, and I'm still amazed at how effective it is, especially in the areas of diet, exercise and health." — Jon Lovgren, author of *The Magic Words: The Pathway to Peace, Joy, and Happiness Where Miracles Become Expectations.*

Normally I tell my clients that change takes time. However, using this prayer on a daily basis every time a negative emotional addiction comes up will quicken your journey toward a body you love! Practice this prayer daily, and it will change your life!

Practice: Ho'oponopono

Say this prayer to yourself. Put your hands on your heart and say,

"I'm sorry…"

I'm sorry for becoming emotionally addicted to frustration, hopelessness, anger, jealousy and all the negative emotions that have kept me in a body I don't love for so long. I'm sorry for making the emotional frequency of not feeling good enough normal in my body.

I'm sorry for creating negative emotions about myself that are so strong I can't even look in the mirror or have my picture taken without feeling insecure, frustrated and unattractive. I'm sorry for allowing the feeling of not being lovable to feel normal to me.

I'm sorry that my soul needed to go through experiences that created self-loathing and pain in my heart to show me where I need to focus the love inside me.

"Please forgive me…"

Forgive me for continuing to hold these frequencies in my body and wanting to give up. Forgive me for not practicing a new way of being.

Forgive me for not having compassion for myself for everything I've been through in life. Forgive me for not giving myself a break and loving all the parts that make me, me.

"Thank you…"

Thank you for the experiences that have shown me what I need to work on to have peace and happiness in my life. Thank you that I'm always taken care of in ways I know and in ways I don't know.

Thank you that my heart beats without me thinking about it and my lungs breathe on their own. Thank you for all the processes and systems in my body that happen for me to live in this human body and be alive.

Thank you, Universe, for always sending me unconditional love even if I can't feel it.

"I love you…"

I love you for being brave enough to take this human experience. I love you for going through challenging times and surviving them in the best way you knew how.

I love you for giving me so many amazing experiences and more to come. I love knowing that I can live in a body I love and am excited to have that experience. I love knowing the Universe is constantly sending me love at all times, just the way I am.

Practice this prayer daily whenever you feel a negative thought come up. If this is all you take with you from this book, it will be enough.

Healing Society

The reason so many people struggle with self-love and experience dieting hell is because, as a society, we've unconsciously created it as part of our ideology. I touched briefly on this in the prior chapter. This is how we've created our self-loathing ideology together...

Magazines show photoshopped models that are supposed to represent what is beautiful. It's unrealistic, and in my opinion, cruel. As a society, we've allowed it to be okay to exploit women's bodies and say that things like cellulite, which is a natural part of maturing skin, is ugly. Social ideology changes all the time. A few hundred years ago, society believed that being overweight was beautiful because people didn't have enough to eat, and if you were overweight, it meant you had wealth.

Ideology not only affects your self-image but also different circumstances in the world. I once heard Marianne Williamson speak and someone asked her, "If our thoughts create our reality, why are there starving children in the world? Are they thinking negatively?"

I will never forget her answer. She simply said, "There are starving children in the world not because they are thinking negatively but because we are."

This is the same reason so many women struggle with weight and body image. If we all felt that a woman's body is beautiful as it ages, with cellulite, larger thighs, droopy skin and a poochy belly, you would feel more self-love and I probably wouldn't have written this book.

You can use Ho'oponopono to not only heal yourself, but help heal society of our current ideology and move it toward more love, acceptance, forgiveness and peace.

Ho'oponopono Story

Here is an example of a man who healed an entire ward of the criminally insane using Ho'oponopono only on himself. Dr. Ihaleakala Hew Len, an expert in the spiritual practice of Ho'oponopono, was asked to help a Hawaii state hospital where the mentally insane patients were totally out of control.[36]

He worked for three years but didn't once see or counsel a single patient. All he did was review their files and practice Ho'oponopono on himself, taking one hundred percent responsibility for how he was experiencing the patient and healing that part inside himself. By the end of three years, the hospital closed because all the patients were healed!

When asked how this was possible, Dr. Len said, "The question is what is going on in me that I'm experiencing this per-

---

[36] Patrice C. (2018). The true story of how one man healed insane patients by working on himself – Ho'oponopono [Article]. Retrieved from http://healingearth.info/hooponopono/

son or situation this way. When I let it go in me, the person or situation gets better."

I had to rewrite this chapter many times because it took me a while to fully grasp what he's talking about, and when I got it, it blew my mind! Dr. Len believes that every experience you have is happening through a shared mind of universal consciousness. If a person is behaving poorly and you are there experiencing it, then it is showing you the part of you out of alignment with love. The situation is in your life to reveal what needs to be healed inside of you.

Isn't that beautiful?

Amazon Story

When I was researching this information, I had an experience where I got to practice Ho'oponopono. I wanted to return something on Amazon that cost $140. The seller only wanted to give me ten percent back and have me sell the product on Amazon myself.

My first response was anger, annoyance, feeling insulted and frustrated. However, I was in the middle of learning this work, so I thought to myself… if this is happening, there is something inside me coming up to be healed. I thought of the times I lived in scarcity and felt disappointment, which I'm sure this person felt when I wanted to return their item.

I said Ho'oponopono to myself:

"I'm sorry there is a misalignment in me that has created this experience.

I ask forgiveness from myself for this misalignment.

I choose to re-align with love for myself and others so I can see the perfection and wholeness in this guy from Amazon.

Thank you for showing me what I need to heal in myself that will bring more joy and peace to our planet."

OMG! The feeling of peace that immediately came over me was overwhelming. I knew everything was going to work out with the Amazon guy, and it did! I got a full refund and things went very smoothly.

I want to say this again so it's really clear: It's not that you're blaming yourself for what others are doing. It's that you're healing the part of you that is ready to be healed and the situation is showing you what that is. It's simply about healing parts of you not lined up with love.

When Dr. Len was brought to the hospital to help the patients and he did Ho'oponopono on himself, he wasn't blaming himself for the people being insane and out of control. He was healing the part of his consciousness that created **his experience** of the mentally insane patients being out of control.

Every human being is whole and complete, and since he was experiencing something other than that, there was something in his consciousness that was out of alignment with love and needed to be healed, and that's why he was having that experience.

When he healed that part of himself, the person or experience moved toward love and got better. It's like what Dr. Wayne Dyer said…

"Change the way you look at things and the things you look at change."

This practice says that you are not a victim in your life. You're a creator and a healer of yourself and others. I LOVE THIS! I can't describe the amount of peace this work brings into your life when you truly practice it. Again, if this is the only thing you do out of this whole book, it will be enough.

I want to tell you my personal prayer. Since I am experiencing a world where many women do not love themselves just the way they are, there must be something inside me that needs to be healed.

My Ho'oponopono Prayer

I'm sorry…

I'm sorry that there is a misalignment in me that has created a lack of self-love in the world.

I'm sorry I've judged my body and others, based on what I've seen on TV, in movies and in magazines.

I'm sorry that I've criticized my legs, arms, breasts and belly and left myself feeling unlovable, and that misalignment has created a lack of self-love that so many others have for their own bodies.

Please forgive me…

I ask forgiveness from myself for being misaligned and believing that my body isn't beautiful just the way it is.

I ask forgiveness from myself for judging other women and not seeing them as unique and beautiful just the way they are.

Thank you…

Thank you, Universe, for showing me this misalignment so it may be healed and have a ripple effect to the dear souls reading this book and around the world.

I love you…

I send love to myself that I may feel peace, full self-acceptance and have that energy extend to the far corners of the planet.

I am so grateful for the unconditional love of the Universe that is always with me even when I can't feel it.

Together we can create a new ideology of love and peace, and we do it by first healing ourselves.

It's not a mistake you're reading this. I visualized that my book would find its way to people who need it and were ready to learn this information, and it's in your hands. You found this book to bring forth a new version of yourself that lives in a body you love. It's what you wanted for so long and it's what you're meant to experience!

I hope by now you realize that living in a body you love doesn't mean you're a size 4! It starts with understanding your emotional addictions, acknowledging and fully accepting all you've been through with compassion for yourself, letting your heart feel love and joy, and bringing forgiveness, love and peace to the parts of you that feel dark and painful. Lastly, eating in a way that leaves you feeling good in your body and about yourself. Only then can you end dieting hell!

You can do this! It's time. It's what you were born to do! When you are living in a body you love, the world becomes a better place for all of us.

Thank you for reading this book. You don't have to live in frustration, hopelessness and shame. It's time to have peace and to release the weight. You deserve that!

Your Fitness and Weight Release Ally,

Michelle

About the Author

Michelle Melendez has been a group exercise instructor since 1996, when she helped open the first aerobics and fitness gym for women in San Luis Obispo, California. At that time, she also became a personal trainer and in 2009 she got her weight-loss specialist certifications.

She is certified to teach many different kinds of exercise classes, including: Body Pump, Reebok Spin, Martial Fitness Kick-boxing, Bosu, Senior Balance, the Pilates Method, R.I.P.P.E.D., and more!

Michelle founded the Pilates Cardiocamp, now Pilates Full-Body, in 2001 in Los Altos, California, and founded Women Being Fit in 2007, an online business teaching women around the world how to live in a body they love.

Michelle currently made her dream of a one hundred percent online fitness business happen in January 2019 when she moved to the Big Island of Hawaii. Clients in her *Live in a Body You Love* program join her twice a year for a week-long healing retreat where she takes them swimming with dolphins, snorkeling with manta rays, hiking the volcano, and more.

Engage with Michelle at **www.womenbeingfit.com**, or call: 866.339.4438. Join her community on Facebook at **facebook.com/womenbeingfit/**

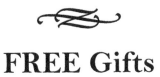

FREE Gifts

Live in a Body You Love Video Series:
WomenBeingFit.com/BodyYouLove

Burn Your Fat, Free Your Heart Cardio practice:
WomenBeingFit.com/BurnFatCardio

Tone Your Body, Lift Your Mood
Strength Training Workout:
WomenBeingFit.com/FunWorkout

Discover how to train for your body type by visiting:
WomenBeingFit.com/FitnessQuiz

Does your body need a detox?
Find out here: WomenBeingFit.com/DetoxQuiz

To book Michelle to speak to your group
or to interview her, please go to …
WomenBeingFit.com/Speaker

Coming Soon by Michelle Melendez

Live In A Body You Love Year-Long Calendar
A year-long calendar with daily inspirations taken from
Michelle's Live in a Body You Love 90-Day program.

God Whispers
Short-stories of intuitive choices that led to
meaningful connections and experiences.

Wahine
A story of strength, spiritual awakening, a
Hawaiian adventure and more!
(Based on a true story.)

Be the first to get your copy visit:
WomenBeingFit.com/NewBooks

Books Michelle Recommends

31-Day Food Revolution: Heal Your Body, Feel Great and Transform Your World by Ocean Robbins

Breaking the Habit of Being Yourself: How to Lose Your Mind and Create a New One" by Joe Dispenza and Daniel G. Amen

Never Be Sick Again: One Disease, Two Causes, Six Pathways by Raymond Francis

The Magic Words: The Pathway to Peace, Joy, and Happiness Where Miracles Become Expectations by Jon Lovgren

Cited Sources in Alphabetical Order

"5 Benefits of Starting Your Day With Himalayan Salt Water (Sole Water)," by NDTV Food Desk, (2018). [Article]. Retrieved from https://food.ndtv.com/food-drinks/5-benefits-of-starting-your-day-with-himalayan-salt-water-sole-water-1728441

"Addictive Heart Energy," by Dr. Bradley Nelson, (2019). [Article]. Retrieved from https://www.healingconsciousness.co.uk/addictive-heart-energy/

"A World Without Cancer (HQ) – The Story of Vitamin B17," by. G. Edward Griffin, (2012). [Documentary]. Retrieved from https://www.youtube.com/watch?v=sKhzbcpI_ro&t=107s

"Breaking the Habit of Being Yourself: How to Lose Your Mind and Create a New One," by Joe Dispenza and Daniel G. Amen, Hay House, 2015.

"Characterizing the Effect of the Energy Emitted by Trinfinity8 on Human DNA," by Dr. Glen Rein, (2012). [Study]. Retrieved from https://www.trinfinity8.com/research-dr-glen-rein/

"Dr. Mercola and Dr. Pickering Discuss Food Combining," by Dr. Mercola (2013). [Video Interview]. Retrieved from https://www.youtube.com/watch?v=fS8PY0RQcNw&t=75s

"Electrophysiological Evidence of Intuition: Part 2. A System-Wide Process," By McCraty, Rollin; Atkinson, Mike; and Bradley, Raymond Trevor. (2004). [Article]. Retrieved from https://www.liebertpub.com/doi/10.1089/107555304323062310

"Fat Grams – How Much Fat Should You Eat Per Day?" By Franziska Spritzler, RD, CDE, (2016). [Article]. Retrieved from https://www.healthline.com/nutrition/how-much-fat-to-eat

Fed Up. Dir. Stephanie Soechtig. 2014. Film.

"Full-Spectrum Cancer Therapy: an interview with James Forsythe," by the Healing Matrix with Regina Meredith. (2013). [Video Interview]. Gaiam TV Original Episode.

"Heart Intelligence: The Heart Is More Powerful Than the Brain – Gregg Braden & Howard Martin," by Scott Helton. (2018). [Article]. Retrieved from https://cafenamaste.com/heart-intelligence-more-powerful-than-brain-gregg-braden/

"Laughter is the Best Medicine," by Lawrence Robinson, Melinda Smith, M.A., and Jeanne Segal, Ph.D. (2018). [Article]. Retrieved from https://www.helpguide.org/articles/mental-health/laughter-is-the-best-medicine.htm/

"Leading Cancer Cases and Deaths, Male and Female," United States Cancer Statistics. (2015). [Statistics]. Retrieved from https://gis.cdc.gov/Cancer/USCS/DataViz.html

"Nation's Largest Health Care Organization Wants to Make Plant-Based Diets the New Normal," By Michael Greger, M.D. (2016). [Article]. Retrieved from https://foodrevolution.org/blog/food-and-health/plant-based-diets-the-new-normal/

"Never Be Sick Again: One Disease, Two Causes, Six Pathways," by Raymond Francis, M.Sc. Health Communications Inc. (2002).

"Plant-Based Diets as the Nutritional Equivalent of Quitting Smoking," by Michael Greger M.D. FACLM. (2017). [Article]. Retrieved from https://nutritionfacts.org/2017/08/01/plant-based-diets-as-the-nutritional-equivalent-of-quitting-smoking/

"Plant-Based Protein: What You Need to Know," Ocean Robbins. (2019). [Article]. Retrieved from https://foodrevolution.org/blog/plant-based-protein/

"Sugar Science, How Much Is Too Much? The growing concern over too much added sugar in our diets," by Sugar

Science. [Article]. Retrieved from http://sugarscience.ucsf.
edu/the-growing-concern-of-overconsumption.html#.
XPHcEi2ZPyI

"Sunlight — It Does Your Body Good," by Dr. Mercola.
(2015). [Article]. Retrieved from https://articles.mercola.
com/sites/articles/archive/2015/12/27/vitamin-d-sunlight.
aspx

"The Answer to Cancer: an Interview with Dr. Leonard
Coldwell," by *Beyond Belief with George Noory*. (2013).
[Video Interview]. Gaiam TV Original Episode.

"The Emotion Code: How to Release Your Trapped Emotions
for Abundant Health, Love and Happiness," by Dr. Bradley
Nelson, Wellness Unmasked, 2011.

"The Little Soul and the Sun," (A Children's Parable Adopted
From Conversations With God) by Neale Donald Walsch,
Hampton Roads, 1998.

"The Recommended Intake of Grams of Carbohydrates
per Day for Women." by Erin Coleman, R.D., L.D.
(2018). [Article]. Retrieved from https://healthyeat-
ing.sfgate.com/recommended-intake-grams-carbohy-
drates-per-day-women-5883.html

"The surprising dangers of CT scans and X-rays," by
Consumer Reports, (2015). [Article] Retrieved from https://

www.consumerreports.org/cro/magazine/2015/01/the-sur-prising-dangers-of-ct-sans-and-x-rays/index.htm

"The true story of how one man healed insane patients by working on himself – Ho'oponopono," by Patrice C. (2018). [Article]. Retrieved from http://healingearth.info/hooponopono/

"The Untethered Soul: the Journey Beyond Yourself," by Michael A. Singer, New Harbinger, 2007.

"Vitamin D may protect against cancer," by Jasmin Collier. (2018). [Article]. Retrieved from https://www.medicalnewstoday.com/articles/321151.php

"Your Soul Contract Decoded: Discovering the Spiritual Map of Your Life with Numerology," by Nicolas David Ngan, New York: Osprey Publishing, 2013.

Resources

"Absolute Perfection! Your Complete Program for a Slim, Lean Waistline (an amazing body too!)" by the editors of Oxygen, Robert Kennedy Publishing, 2007.

"7 Benefits of Complex Carbs and the Best Ones to Eat," by Heather McCless. (2017). [Article]. Retrieved from https://www.onegreenplanet.org/vegan-food/benefits-of-complex-carbs-and-the-best-ones-to-eat/

"7 Impressive Ways Vitamin C Benefits Your Body," by Ryan Raman, MS, RD. (2018). [Article]. Retrieved from https://www.healthline.com/nutrition/vitamin-c-benefits

"8 Non-Toxic Cookware Brands to Keep Chemicals Out of Your Food," by Emily Monaco. (2019). [Article]. Retrieved from http://www.organicauthority.com/7-non-toxic-cookware-brands-to-keep-chemicals-out-of-your-food/

"10 Science-Backed Reasons to Eat More Protein," by Kris Gunnars, BSc. (2019). [Article]. Retrieved from https://www.healthline.com/nutrition/10-reasons-to-eat-more-protein

"An Immunity Booster Against Cancer and Aging?" By Marion Tible, PhD. (2018). [Article]. Retrieved from http://www.longlonglife.org/en/transhumanism-longevity/anti-aging-supplements/ip6-immunity-booster-against-cancer-anti-aging/

"Are You Addicted to Suffering and Struggle?" By Anderson, Anna (2016). [Article]. Retrieved from https://www.huffpost.com/entry/are-you-addicted-to-suffe_b_9744416

"Becoming Supernatural: How Common People Are Doing the Uncommon," by Dr. Dispenza, Joe. Carlsbad: Hay House, Inc. 2012

"Essiac Tea: Ingredients, Benefits and Side Effects," by Rachael Link, MS, RD. (2018). [Article]. Retrieved from https://www.healthline.com/nutrition/essiac-tea#anticancer-benefits

"Electrophysiological Evidence of Intuition: Part 2. A System-Wide Process," by McCraty, Rollin; Atkinson, Mike; and Bradley, Raymond Trevor. (2004). [Article]. Retrieved from https://www.liebertpub.com/doi/10.1089/107555304323062310

"Food Choices Change Our Gene Expression," by Dr. David Perlmutter. (2015). [Article]. Retrieved from https://www.drperlmutter.com/food-choices-change-gene-expression/

"Food is Information: An Interview with Dr. Christiane Northrup," by Dr. Mark Hyman MD. (2016). [Video

Interview]. Retrieved from https://drhyman.com/blog/2016/09/30/food-is-information-an-interview-with-dr-christiane-northrup/

"Glutathione and Cancer," by Dr. Véronique Desaulniers. (2016). [Article]. Retrieved from https://www.beatcancer.org/blog-posts/glutathione-and-cancer

"High-Dose Vitamin C (PDQ®)–Health Professional Version," by Nagi B. Kumar, PhD, RD, FADA; and Jeffrey D. White, MD. (2019). [Article]. Retrieved from https://www.cancer.gov/about-cancer/treatment/cam/hp/vitamin-c-pdq

"Integrating Poly-MVA into protocols for cancer, degenerative disease, and other health challenges," by Cancer Tutor. (2019). [Article]. Retrieved from https://www.cancertutor.com/poly-mva/

"Let Your Heart Talk to Your Brain," by HeartMath LLC, Contributor. (2013). [Article]. Retrieved from https://www.huffpost.com/entry/heart-wisdom_n_2615857

"National Cancer Institute Drug Dictionary," [Synopsis]. Retrieved from https://www.cancer.gov/publications/dictionaries/cancer-drug/def/green-tea-extract

"Tap water Toxins," by HappyPreppers.com (2019). [Article]. Retrieved from http://www.happypreppers.com/tapwater.html

"The Great American Health Hoax: the Surprising Truth About How Modern Medicine Keeps You Sick," by Francis, Raymon. Deerfield Beach: Health Communications, Inc. 2014

"The Effects of Stress on Your Body," by Ann Pietrangelo and Stephanie Watson (2017). [Article]. Retrieved from https://www.healthline.com/health/stress/effects-on-body#1

"The Heart's Electromagnetic Field" by information-book. com, [Article]. Retrieved from: http://www.information-book. com/biology-medicine/biofields-heart-electromagnetic-field/

"The Recommended Intake of Grams of Carbohydrates per Day for Women," by Erin Coleman, R.D., L.D. (2018). [Article]. Retrieved from https://healthyeating.sfgate.com/recommended-intake-grams-carbohydrates-per-day-women-5883.html

"Vitamin D may protect against cancer," by Honor Whiteman, (2018). [Article]. Retrieved from https://www.medicalnewstoday.com/articles/321151.php.

"Vitamin D2 vs. D3: What's the Difference?" By Atli Arnarson, PhD., (2018). [Article]. Retrieved from https://www.healthline.com/nutrition/vitamin-d2-vs-d3

"Resveratrol and Cancer," by Andrea S. Blevins Primeau, PhD, MBA. (2018). [Article]. Retrieved from https://

www.cancertherapyadvisor.com/home/tools/fact-sheets/resveratrol-and-cancer/

"Why Essiac Tea Should be Part of Your Cancer Fighting Program," by Dr. David Jockers, DC, MS, CSCS. (2015). [Article] Retrieved from https://thetruthaboutcancer.com/essiac-tea-cancer-fighting/

"What Happens to Your Body When You Eat Too Much Sugar?" by Dr. Mercola. (2019). [Article]. Retrieved from https://articles.mercola.com/sugar-side-effects.aspx.

"Why Is Water Important? 16 Reasons to Drink Up," by Natalie Butler, RD, LD. (2019). [Article]. Retrieved from https://www.healthline.com/health/food-nutrition/why-is-water-important#digestion

Made in the USA
Middletown, DE
13 June 2020